The story of Dr. Sidney R. Garfield

The Story of **Dr. Sidney R. Garfield**

The Visionary Who Turned
Sick Care into Health Care

TOM DEBLEY

IN COLLABORATION WITH
JON STEWART

The Permanente Press
Oakland, California • Portland, Oregon

About the Authors:

Tom Debley is Director of Heritage Resources for Kaiser Permanente. Trained originally as a journalist, he had a career as an award-winning reporter for many years before moving into public affairs and history work. He has worked on significant historical research and related communication projects for the University of California in addition to Kaiser Permanente.

Jon Stewart is Director of Communications for Government Relations and Health Policy at Kaiser Permanente and an editor of *The Permanente Journal*. Following a long career in daily journalism, he joined Kaiser Permanente as the first communications director for The Permanente Federation, the umbrella organization for all the Permanente Medical Groups, on whose behalf he has championed the history and the promise of Permanente Medicine.

Cover:
The painting of Dr. Sidney Garfield by St. John Moran hangs in the Board Room of The Permanente Medical Group in Oakland, California.

© 2009 by The Permanente Press

Published 2009 by The Permanente Press
Oakland, California • Portland, Oregon

The Permanente Press is owned by The Permanente Federation, LLC
Oakland, California

THE STORY OF DR. SIDNEY R. GARFIELD
THE VISIONARY WHO TURNED SICK CARE INTO HEALTH CARE

20 19 18 17 16   6 7 8 9

ISBN: 978-0-9770463-2-4
Library of Congress Control Number: 2008944214

Book design by Lynette Leisure
Printed in the United States of America

Dedicated to the
tens of thousands of
Permanente physicians
who have followed
in the wake of
Sidney R. Garfield, M.D.

❧ Table of Contents ❧

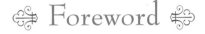

Foreword

The Lasting Legacy of
Sidney R. Garfield, M.D.

By Jay Crosson, M.D.

It's about time. For too long, Sidney Garfield, M.D., has stood in the giant shadow cast by his more celebrated partner and friend, Henry J. Kaiser, the great entrepreneur and industrialist. Mr. Kaiser's name and fame live on, mainly in association with the only nonprofit organization ever incorporated by the builder of more than 100 for-profit companies — Kaiser Permanente. But the physician whose extraordinary vision and daring innovations in health care delivery gave birth to that same organization remains largely unrecognized beyond the select circle of medical historians and the heritage-minded physicians and staff of Kaiser Permanente.

One needn't minimize the vital role of Mr. Kaiser in Kaiser Permanente's story to assert the seminal role played by Dr. Garfield. They were genuine partners, each bringing to the enterprise critical elements lacking in the other: money and organizational genius from Mr. Kaiser; a visionary mind and an unrelenting drive for innovation and quality improvement from Dr. Garfield; and from both a genuine belief in and commitment to human dignity and progress.

The recent centennial of Dr. Garfield's birth in 1906 provides a timely occasion not only to recall and celebrate his role in creating and evolving the unique model of health care delivery that would become Kaiser Permanente, but to examine as well some of his key insights and innovations with regard to the current and future state of American health care.

Anyone who has examined Dr. Garfield's long career will appreciate the difficulty of assessing the historical and/or current relevance of his ideas and innovations. As his diminishing number of surviving colleagues will attest, he was a fount of ideas — virtual intellectual fireworks — admittedly igniting a few duds among the brilliant rockets. The ideas ranged across the entire spectrum of health care, from delivery models to financing to hospital design. In the end, it may fairly be said that he achieved his childhood dream of becoming an engineer (he is said to have broken down and cried when his parents insisted he attend medical school) by engineering our unique model of health care.

But among all his many lasting contributions, which ones constitute the essential core of his life's work? And what relevance do they have for today and tomorrow?

I believe Dr. Garfield's lasting reputation will rest on four big ideas that, individually and in combination, powered fundamental transformations in health care. They are:

- the change from fee-for-service to prepayment;
- the promotion of multispecialty group practice in combination with prepayment;
- the emphasis on prevention and early detection to accomplish what he termed "the new economy of medicine," in which providers would be rewarded for keeping people healthy; and,
- finally — and most presciently — the centrality of information technology in the future of health care.

Significantly, each one of these 20th century innovations, three of which are deeply embedded in Kaiser Permanente's own genetic code, is at or near a critical crossroads in this first decade of the 21st century, as the nation considers its options for redesigning the American health care system. Let us briefly examine each in turn.

Prepayment

In his work, in the 1930s, at his little fee-for-service Contractors General Hospital in the Mojave Desert caring for aqueduct construction workers, Dr. Garfield was saved from the looming threat of bankruptcy by the discovery of prepayment to the delivery system for comprehensive services. The idea was borrowed from the Ross-Loos Clinic in Los Angeles County and was rooted in the late 19th century traditions of "industrial medicine." Collecting a dime a day from approximately 5,000 aqueduct workers, Dr. Garfield's desert office and small hospital prospered under prepayment, and his eyes were opened to the transformation of care made possible when wellness rather than sickness became a revenue source.

Prepayment, he said, "is the old principle of the well paying for the sick; the houses that don't burn down paying for those that do."[1] But even more important, he noted, prepayment "brings the patient to the doctor earlier in his illness and more often, which is one of the most important effects … because it permits the practice of true preventive medicine. Any plan that sets a barrier between the patient and the doctor by eliminating the first two or three visits, by covering the patient only for hospital or surgical care, or by limiting this coverage in other ways, in our opinion defeats its purpose and is not good."[1]

Employer-based prepayment led Dr. Garfield inevitably to a focus on prevention and what would come to be known as health maintenance and wellness. It solved for him the critical question of the economics of medicine: "how to keep the people of this country well and healthy and, at the same time, preserve the medical and hospital organization which must do that job, but under our present (fee-for-service) system derives its income out of sickness."[1]

Prepayment for comprehensive services has served as one of the critical strands of Kaiser Permanente's DNA since the very beginning of the organization when Dr. Garfield first partnered with Mr. Kaiser to provide employee health services at Grand Coulee Dam and later in the World War II shipyards. Yet 60 years later, in an era of industry-wide cost-shifting and a proliferation of high-deductible plans, we are confronting a question that Dr. Garfield might have found unthinkable: Would Kaiser Permanente still be Kaiser Permanente without prepayment?

The principle of prepayment for comprehensive services is challenged today, primarily because the growing cost of health coverage has pushed employers to favor insurance plans with high deductibles and to move toward self insurance. Each of these is to some degree in conflict with the concept of prepaid, comprehensive benefits that have long been a defining feature of Kaiser Permanente.

High deductible plans create financial disincentives for patients to seek preventive services and can lead patients to forego coordinated office-based care for chronic diseases such as hypertension and diabetes. What is the right balance between unfettered, out-of-pocket personal liability for health care and open-ended social insurance? Kaiser Permanente, as well as those seeking to design the best model for national universal health coverage are struggling with this question at this time. In the long run, there is good reason to believe Kaiser Permanente can and will adapt to the market and to health care reform by developing more intelligent and clinically sound cost-sharing benefit designs without creating significant barriers to needed care. Such work is currently under way under the term "value-based benefit design."

Multispecialty Group Practice

With the financial security provided by prepayment, Dr. Garfield was able to realize his second great contribution to what would become Permanente Medicine — multispecialty group practice. Here again the idea was not unique to Dr. Garfield, but borrowed from other pioneers, such as the Mayo brothers in Minnesota and, especially, Dr. Garfield's own experience with a form of group practice at Los Angeles County General Hospital. There he had served as a chief resident with other first generation Permanente physicians, including Wallace Neighbor, M.D., (first Medical Director of what would become Northwest Permanente) and Raymond Kay, M.D., (founding Medical Director of the Southern California Permanente Medical Group). "We grew up at the county hospital," was how Dr. Garfield put it.[1]

"It has always seemed a paradox," said Dr. Garfield in later life, "that in universities, which teach us medicine, we learn medicine under the highest type of group practice, but when we go out into practice, we revert to the old type of individual private practice."[1]

Dr. Garfield's great contribution to the evolution of group practice was to layer onto it the additional power of two other elements: prepayment and integration of the medical group with what he termed "adequate facilities" — "bringing the doctors' offices, laboratory, X-ray, and hospital ... all together under one roof."[1] Group practice alone could be a powerful engine for continuous learning and coordination of care; integrating it with the full range of medical facilities served to align the otherwise conflicting interests of doctors and hospitals; and then layering on prepayment removed financial barriers to care while opening the door to prevention and health maintenance. With all these elements in synergistic combination — first achieved at Dr. Garfield's Mason City Hospital at Grand Coulee Dam, where Mr. Kaiser first saw and embraced Dr. Garfield's vision — the young surgeon, still in his mid-30s, had engineered the miracle of Permanente Medicine.

Over the past 60 years, the Permanente Medical Groups, which evolved out of the old Garfield and Associates, have been more successful than any group in the country at exploiting and enriching the possibilities of multispecialty group practice — largely because of the grafting on of prepayment and integrated facilities, as well as our sustaining partnership with Kaiser Foundation Health Plan and a tradition of great physician leadership and professionalism. This unique model has set the standards for both efficiency and clinical quality in most of the communities in which we operate, and it continues to be touted by some of the smartest minds in the country (and not all within Permanente) as the best solution to the multiple crises besetting American health care.

And yet, 74 years after the National Committee on the Costs of Medical Care advocated group practice as "essential" to "meet the modern demands of medical science and technology,"[2] group practices still occasionally have to defend this style of practice against the tradition of solo and small group practice. What's more, it is facing significant challenges from the concept of so-called "high-performance networks," an insurance-company driven promise of "groups without walls" — and, in most cases, without clinical coordination or any form of economic integration.

Given the disaggregated nature of the delivery system in most communities today, insurers have been able to promote the idea that they can achieve all the advantages of an actual group practice by profiling individual doctors and hospitals, selecting the most efficient providers, and then lumping them all together into a pseudo-systemic "high-performing network" with an external stand-alone disease management component. In a world that still clings tenaciously to Marcus Welby, M.D., it looks to some like a reasonable alternative to genuine group practice. However, performance measurement systems such as the HEDIS measurements of the National Committee for Quality Assurance (NCQA), and academic studies such as that by Gillies, et. al.,[3] show clearly that group practice-based care produces better results for patients.

Prevention

As I have noted, preventive health care and health promotion became an early principle of Permanente Medicine as a direct result of prepayment, which put a premium on keeping workers (and, later, whole communities) healthy. Recalling his early experience with prepayment in the Mojave Desert, Dr. Garfield noted that the "financial result (of prepayment) was impressive, but another result impressed us very much — a resulting change in our attitude. Prior to (prepayment), we were anxious to have injured workers come into the hospital, since it meant remuneration … Under the new arrangement, we had the same amount of income whether the workers were injured or not. Obviously, we were better off if they remained unhurt."[1] And thus began Dr. Garfield's long and growing interest in safety engineering, preventive health, and health education and wellness programs.

The great tradition and growing sophistication of preventive medicine at Kaiser Permanente since Dr. Garfield's time would, I am certain, impress and gratify him. Motivated by awareness that preventable illness makes up 70 percent or more of the total burden of illness and its associated costs, Kaiser Permanente has long embraced an expanding concept of prevention and early detection of disease that includes, in addition to such traditional practices as immunizations and periodic screenings, a broad array of health promotion and patient self-management practices. Through the Care Management Institute and our research units, we have focused on the development and diffusion of evidence-based guidelines for preventive practices and self-care for patients with chronic and complex conditions. And with the implementation of our KP HealthConnect electronic medical record, we are now capable of driving the promises of preventive medicine to an entirely new level of practice, with automated physician reminders and an array of patient-oriented health education and self-management tools.

The concept of preventive care has also had great impacts across the entire health care environment. Most of the NCQA-HEDIS measures by which health care organizations are evaluated for clinical quality are actually preventive and early detection practices, as are many of the measures by which health plans and providers will be reimbursed in most of the new pay-for-performance initiatives.

However, as health care costs continue to push against the limits of middle-class affordability, the importance of many preventive practices is losing ground in some significant ways.

As we know from our own research, whereas some common preventive practices may be cost effective at an employer or social level (by reducing absenteeism, for instance), they may not be for the health care industry in isolation. This fact has led some insurers to underpay primary care physicians for preventive services. The result has been a threatened shortage of primary care physicans coming out of American medical schools. Hopefully the emergence of the "medical home" idea as a basis for enhanced payment for primary care coordination will begin to reverse this trend.

Further, as noted above, early evidence from the introduction of high-deductible health plans in the U. S. suggests lower compliance with needed visits and medications for patients with chronic conditions such as diabetes and hypertension.

Information Technology

Were Sidney Garfield to make an appearance today, I suspect he would be aghast that so many other aspects of American life and work have enjoyed the benefits of sophisticated information systems while large portions of the health care industry remain largely stuck in the Paper Age. Having envisioned and promoted many of the great improvements that computers could bring to medicine back in the 1960s, Dr. Garfield — never a patient man — would no doubt wonder why, more than four decades later, it is still not universal, and may require federal legislation and funding to be achieved.

As early as 1960, Dr. Garfield embraced the idea that computers — those giant punch-card machines of the period — could somehow lead to a fundamental transformation of health care delivery. He assigned the brilliant young physician Morris Collen, M.D., an internist who had a degree in electrical engineering, to look into the possibilities. As John Smillie, M.D., recounted in his history of The Permanente Medical Group, Collen reported back "to confirm that Dr. Garfield was correct: Medical electronics was beginning a period of great innovation and diffusion, and … we should begin to take advantage of the potential of electronic digital computers."[4] Remember, this was 1960.

The story of Kaiser Permanente's pioneering work with information technology under the sponsorship of Dr. Garfield and the direction of Dr. Collen is a remarkable tale. Not more than half a dozen places in the world were doing comparable research in health care. As early as 1968, Dr. Garfield could confidently write that "the computer cannot replace the physician, but it can keep essential data moving smoothly from laboratory to nurse's station, from X-ray department to the patient's chart, and from all areas of the medical center to the physician himself."[1] Two years earlier, Dr. Collen had declared in a speech to the Minnesota State Medical Association that "the computer will probably have the greatest impact on medical science since the invention of the microscope."[1]

By 1970, when Dr. Garfield spelled out his grand vision for the future of medicine in *Scientific American,*[5] he included a series of diagrams of the evolution of health systems through the decades, beginning in 1900. At the center of each diagram up to 1970 was the hospital — the central axis of the system. In his diagram of the system of the future, the hospital is replaced by the "computer center" — an amazingly prescient vision for the time. He began telling his Permanente colleagues that they had all the elements of a "jet-engined plan" for health care, but without the computer and other innovations, such as health education centers and expanded use of nurse practitioners, they remained hitched to a "buggy" of traditional medical practice.

Despite the many fits and starts, leaps and stumbles along the almost half century-long path to KP HealthConnect, I am certain Dr. Garfield would be proud of the organization today for the leadership it has continued to show by implementing the largest and most sophisticated health information technology system in the world at a time when much of American health care is still debating the "business case for IT." Although Dr. Garfield would be on familiar ground with many of the capabilities of KP HealthConnect, he would have to be impressed by at least one major feature: that of rapid, asynchronous two-way communication between doctors and patients, and doctors and doctors, and the ability of patients to input data into their medical record and access information from it. In the pre-Internet era, Drs. Garfield and Collen could only glimpse the full potential of the technology to "virtualize" many elements of the physician-patient relationship, moving much of the interaction downstream in the interests of efficiency and improved service.

Conclusion

As I have noted, the four great ideas on which so much of Dr. Garfield's enduring and future reputation rests are under varying degrees of challenge today. That fact is of legitimate concern to many of us — and to many outside Kaiser Permanente, as well. But perhaps we should also look at these challenges as opportunities — something both Dr. Garfield and Mr. Kaiser were famous for doing. As Dr. Garfield told The Permanente Medical Group executive committee in his annual report in 1964, "Opposition by organized medicine to our program was good for us. It kept us intellectually honest and stimulated us to do better continually."[1]

Just as Dr. Garfield and his fellow Permanente physicians were forced by skeptics and outright powerful opponents to prove the value of group practice and prepayment, the current generation of Permanente doctors and Kaiser Foundation Health Plan leaders and employees are being challenged to bring greater proof of the value of our model to the claims and promises we make to employers and members. In meeting these challenges, we should remember that the principles that Dr. Garfield laid down almost 60 years ago are not so rigid as to be unadaptable to changing realities. In fact they have all evolved in significant ways since they were first articulated. As he warned at an interregional meeting of Permanente physician leaders in 1974: "Institutions tend to become static; they build walls around themselves to protect themselves from change and eventually die. You should fight that [tendency] by opening up your thinking and your ideas, and work for change."[1]

Equally important, however, is the need to understand the contributions of each of these four principles to the evolution of what we have collectively created over the last six decades. We commonly call this Permanente Medicine. The power of prepayment to a multispecialty group practice is, in fact, the engine of Permanente Medicine, an engine that has driven and continually refreshed Kaiser Permanente through good times and bad. We should always strive to preserve and protect the power of this engine.

References

1. Gilford S. Compendium of Quotes. Unpublished manuscript, 2005.

2. Committee on the Costs of Medical Care. Medical Care for the American People: The Final Report of the Committee on the Costs of Medical Care. Chicago: University of Chicago Press, 1932.

3. Gillies R, Chenok KE, Shortell SM, Pawlson G, Wimbush JJ. The impact of health plan delivery system organization on clinical quality and patient satisfaction. HSR: Health Services Research 2006 Aug;41(4) Part 1:1181-99.

4. Smillie J. Can physicians manage the quality and cost of health care? New York: Mcgraw-Hill; 1991.

5. Garfield SR. The delivery of medical care. Sci Am 1970 Apr;222(4):15-23.

Adapted, updated, and edited by Jay Crosson, MD, from The Permanente Journal 2006 Summer, 10(2), Crosson J. Dr. Garfield's Enduring Legacy — Challenges and Opportunities, p 40-5; copyright 2006, with permission from The Permanente Press.

❧ Preface ❧

Henry J. Kaiser is the name most often associated with Kaiser Permanente, the medical care program that was, in his own view, his greatest achievement. He once said, "I only expect to be remembered for … filling the people's greatest need: good health." He also was always careful to acknowledge that he could never have done what he did in health care without his co-founder, surgeon Sidney R. Garfield, M.D.

It was Garfield, starting in the 1930s, who collected three ideas into a single system of medical care: prevention of illness, group medical practice, and facilities under one roof. Garfield advocated for a not-for-profit foundation as the basic financing structure and believed that ideas from academic medical centers — including the linkage of research to care delivery — could be part of a health care program for average patients, not just the elite. In 1938, Henry Kaiser met Garfield for the first time, listened to his ideas, and declared, "Young man, if your ideas are half as good as you say they are, they are good for the entire country."

In 2003, when Kaiser Permanente created the Heritage Resources Department and started its historical archive, there was a manila folder marked "Sidney R. Garfield" with a paltry amount of material, perhaps a quarter inch thick. Fortunately, archivist Bryan Culp soon joined the department and turned that small file into a still-growing mountain of documentary material. Today, our archive holds thousands of pages of Garfield's own words: papers, speeches, interviews, surgical notes, and more. For the first time, a comprehensive collection of invaluable original research material exists about the life, ideas, and contributions of Sidney Garfield.

This book is based upon these collected and reassembled documents — his own and others relating to him. It represents the first time that Garfield's story has been told in a form that puts him in the foreground and Henry Kaiser in the background. This is not, however, a definitive biography — that awaits the work of some future scholar and medical historian. In the following pages I have tried to offer readers a story that provides a comprehensive overview of Garfield's life and contributions. To that end, I chose to use a narrative style uncluttered by footnotes. I am, however, appending a list of works authored and coauthored by Sidney R. Garfield that can be found in the Kaiser Permanente Heritage Archive. These are the specific materials upon which I drew for this story. It is important to point out that every direct quotation in the book is real; I engaged in no literary license. Likewise, every factual statement made here is rooted in one or more reliable historical sources.

Many people deserve thanks for their contributions to this work. Bryan Culp's dedication to finding and archiving materials has, as noted, created the first and only comprehensive collection of Garfield history, now preserved for future research. Steve Gilford, a consulting historian to our archive, spent many years collecting materials and photographs relating to Kaiser Permanente history, often rooting through trash or recycling bins and eBay to salvage and preserve valuable documents. He interviewed scores of individuals with intimate recollections of many of the events recounted here. He also provided excellent commentary and fact-checking on early drafts. Jon Stewart, Communications Director for Government Relations and Health Policy at Kaiser Foundation Health Plan, Inc., deserves special thanks for editing the manuscript, making sense of convoluted passages in the first draft, and for significant rewrites and revisions. Thank you to Max McMillen for editing services and Virginia McPartland for her help with proofreading. Special gratitude goes to the Regional Oral History Office at The Bancroft Library of the University of California at Berkeley, where past and present scholars and oral historians have been documenting the history of Kaiser Permanente. Thank you, too, to Tom Janisse, M.D., publisher of The Permanente Press, for his support.

— Tom Debley, Director, Heritage Resources, Kaiser Permanente

The Desert Doctor

It was an inauspicious beginning — as it would have been for any new physician, let alone a young man of great vision and ambition. The year was 1933, four years into the desperation of the Great Depression. Sidney R. Garfield, having completed his surgical residency at Los Angeles County General Hospital, launched his medical career by leaving the growing metropolis and constructing a compact, 12-bed hospital in the southern end of the desolate Mojave Desert east of Los Angeles, California. His father, Isaac, helped the 27-year-old with a $2,250 loan, about $35,000 in today's dollars. His prosaically named Contractors General Hospital, a mile or so off the then new, two-lane transcontinental U.S. Highway 60, was about halfway between Los Angeles and Phoenix. The nearest town, a roadside outpost called Desert Center, was about six miles to the east. The locale, as described by one observer, was a "hot, dusty region never meant by God for human activity or habitation."

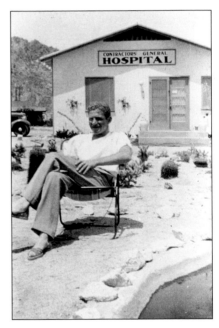

Sidney Garfield at his 12-bed Contractors General Hospital, 1935.

With jobs almost impossible to find, even in medicine, Garfield looked to this remote spot when he learned about construction of the Metropolitan Water District of Southern California's aqueduct designed to bring Colorado River water

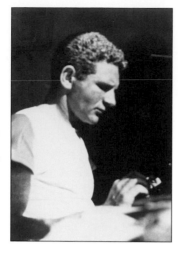

Sidney Garfield catching up on his paperwork at Contractors General Hospital, 1933.

to Los Angeles. Thousands of men were laboring under dangerous and physically demanding conditions in the harsh desert environment. Garfield reasoned they would need on-site medical care.

Desert Center had been founded about a dozen years earlier by an itinerant preacher and cotton farmer at a spot where his car had broken down. It was an aptly named dusty and lonely wide spot on the highway where a traveler could get a meal at the 24-hour café, buy gas, and refill the canvas water bags to use if the car engine overheated while crossing the desert. It was about 50 miles east of Indio, the largest city in the region, where Dr. Gene Morris, former intern at Los Angeles County General Hospital, had grown up and had returned to set up a medical practice. Morris told his friend Garfield about the construction project with thousands of aqueduct workers covered by California's progressive system of workers' compensation, but with no medical or hospital care available near their work camps. The two young doctors formed a partnership and built their wood-frame hospital on the edge of a construction camp. Garfield named it Contractors General Hospital and ensured that it was modern and well-equipped with creature comforts, including air conditioning — an innovation installed in the White House in 1930 but not in widespread use, especially not in rural hospitals.

With 5,000 aqueduct construction workers now at jobsites spread across 150 miles of desert, getting patients, they figured, would not be a problem. The two young doctors were gambling that on-the-job injuries alone would bring them plenty of patients insured for industrial accidents — enough to make the hospital an economic success. They were right. Men suffering from on-the-job injuries did come, but Contractors General tended to get only the relatively minor cases. Insurance companies shipped serious cases — the ones that provided the most significant income — to hospitals in Los Angeles. To make matters worse, the insurance companies discounted the physicians' bills for the care they did give, claiming they over-treated patients. "We got a patient," Garfield explained, "and we would treat him with tender loving care and we would bill the insurance company, and more often than not, they would come back and discount our bills, saying that we treated the patient too many times." Even when the insurance companies did pay, they were slow in paying.

Another problem arose when the aqueduct workers came in with all sorts of illnesses clearly not covered by their workers' compensation insurance, including venereal diseases from prostitutes who also set up shop near the work camps. That would not have been a problem, except that few of the men could pay their medical bills. The cost of treating non-paying patients soon put a major financial strain on the busy little hospital. Discouraged, Dr. Morris sold his share of the partnership to Garfield. Garfield was now on his own, with just one nurse, a housekeeper/cook, and her husband, who served both as orderly and ambulance driver.

As if non-paying patients, slow-paying insurers, rattlesnakes, scorpions, and scorching summer temperatures that rarely dipped below triple digits were not discouragement enough, a new threat to his struggling enterprise arose. One day a sedan turned off Highway 60 in a cloud of dust and headed up the dirt road toward Contractors General. Two men got out and

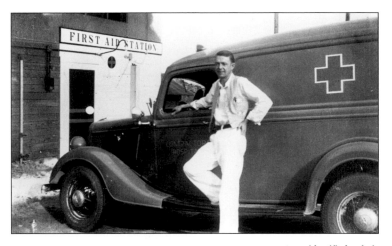

An unidentified orderly standing beside what is believed to be Sidney Garfield's first ambulance.

identified themselves as representatives of a finance company. They had come to seize Garfield's Ford panel truck, which had been outfitted as an ambulance.

Garfield had not been able to afford an ambulance, and a local undertaker in Indio had offered him a deal: He would rent the ambulance to Garfield for $25 a month if Garfield would help him get undertaking work from the aqueduct project. But after more than a year, there had been few deaths. The unhappy undertaker wanted out of the ambulance lease, so he went to a finance company in nearby Riverside, took out a loan using the ambulance as collateral, and then neglected to make the payments. When the finance company complained, he told them to repossess the ambulance.

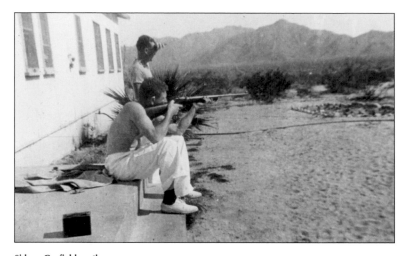

Sidney Garfield on the steps of Contractors General Hospital with the legendary rifle used in the encounter with the ambulance repo men.

Without an ambulance to pick up the sick and injured, the hospital would be out of business. Desperate, Garfield telephoned an attorney-friend in Los Angeles, who called the finance company's attorney. The finance company called off the repo men, who drove away leaving a very relieved Garfield in their dust. The victory was short-lived. The next day, the repo men returned and again demanded the vehicle. Garfield again called his attorney, who said, "No, don't let them do it. They can't take it away." Garfield hung up the phone, went outside, reached through the window of the ambulance and yanked the key out of the ignition. Now unable to start it, the repo men tied a rope to the ambulance's front bumper to tow it away. Garfield slashed the rope with a knife. When they started to retie the rope, Garfield called to a staff member to bring out the rifle they used for recreational target practice.

"Go ahead and shoot," said one of the men defiantly, calculating that a physician would not pull the trigger.

"They had me stumped there," Garfield said later. Instead, he again sliced the rope. Finally, the men left, again without the ambulance. But they reappeared two days later with the county sheriff, who carried a warrant for Garfield's arrest for assault with a deadly weapon. The sheriff, a good friend of Garfield's, explained he had no choice but to take Garfield to jail because of the warrant. His plight had gone from bad to worse. The ambulance was gone, and Garfield, if convicted of assault with a deadly weapon, could lose his medical license.

Fortunately, he rejected his first attorney's advice to plead guilty and pay a fine. With a second attorney, he instead went to trial and won a not-guilty verdict. But being found not guilty was not enough for Garfield, whose honor and reputation were at stake. He sued the undertaker, the finance company, and their attorney for malicious prosecution and won. He was awarded $3,000, a portion of which he promptly used to finance a new ambulance.

The ambulance incident was, in some ways, emblematic of the first phase of Garfield's extraordinary career — the daring desert years of creating something from nothing, of struggling against daunting odds to achieve his ends. Given his determination to succeed, whatever the obstacles, he exhibited a characteristic refusal to allow second thoughts to give him pause. Indeed, Garfield, in these early years, had a vague sense he was working toward something larger than personal success. Today, across the road from old U.S. Highway 60 and the still operating Desert Center Café, where Garfield could celebrate his legal victory with a 50-cent roast beef dinner, stands California Historical Marker No. 992, in Garfield's honor, to announce to occasional visitors that something very special and enduring was born in this lonely corner of the desert.

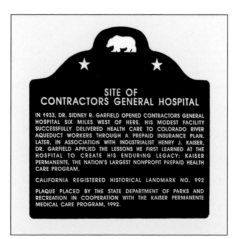

California Historical Marker No. 992 at Desert Center, about six miles east of the site of Contractors General Hospital.

Chapter 1

Out of the Immigrant Forge

Brilliant. Entrepreneurial. Persistent. Stubborn. Self-confident. These are among the traits that served Sidney Garfield well in the difficult, early years of his medical practice, as well as in the later years of creating and realizing his vision. They can be traced from his boyhood, when his parents devoted themselves to preparing him for life in their adopted country. Leaving their home countries with the late 19th and early 20th century emigrants from Eastern Europe and Tsarist Russia, Bertha and Isaac, in 1894, immigrated to the United States where they met and married. Their family names are unknown; Isaac, as frequently happened, adopted a more American-sounding name, Garfield, when he entered the country.

Bertha grew up in a small town not far from Kovno (today's Kaunas), the second largest city in Lithuania. Her father was a local official, and the family was comparatively well-off, enough to afford a servant. But adventurous Bertha was anxious to join her half brother in Chelsea, Massachusetts — a small city near Boston with a large Jewish immigrant population. Isaac came from a more modest background, a peasant family living outside St. Petersburg. He, too, had a brother in Chelsea who welcomed Isaac into his home.

Bertha and Isaac both wanted to become Americans. They took English classes and citizenship courses and may well have met in one of these classes. Isaac began his business life in America peddling household items door-to-door, not an uncommon occupation for a "greenhorn." The work was hard, lugging around a suitcase filled with wares in all kinds of weather. However lowly the work, Isaac saved enough money to open a "gent's furnishing store," as his daughter, Sally, later described it. He set up shop in the port city of Elizabeth, New Jersey, serving laborers, longshoremen, sailors, and their families.

Sidney was born here on April 17, 1906. He and Sally, his older sister, grew up in an apartment above their father's store at 64 First Street. As soon as they were old enough, both children helped out in the store working as salesclerks after school and on weekends. It is likely that this is where young Sidney first learned the sales skills and the value of service that would serve him well in later years.

A good-looking child with his father's striking blue eyes, he embraced Isaac's entrepreneurial spirit and fierce independence. As his father often told him, "It is much better to work for yourself and make $10 than it is to work for someone else for $100."

From his mother, Sidney inherited a shock of red hair that made him the target of taunting by neighborhood bullies to the point that he begged to color his hair.

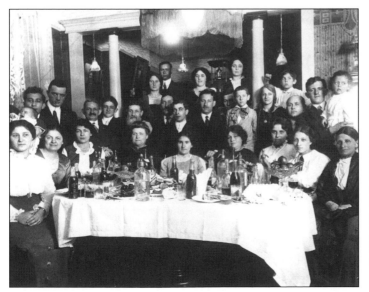

Sidney Garfield with his extended family inside their apartment above his father's store in Elizabeth, New Jersey, around 1914. Eight-year-old Sidney (right-center wearing bow tie) is standing next to his father.

Since good hair dye was not yet in common use, his mother applied a thick black hair cream that dirtied his shirt collars and bed linens. When the barber refused to cut his hair, Bertha escorted her son to the sink and washed out the gooey cream. Sidney learned to live with his red hair, and, as an adult, allowed at least one good friend and colleague to call him "Red."

While Judaism was a part of Sidney's upbringing, it was not of the strict variety. Isaac kept the store open on both Saturday and Sunday, for instance. Sidney had a Bar Mitzvah ceremony on his 13th birthday, marking the crossover from childhood to adulthood, and the family observed Jewish dietary laws at home. But in his adult life, Judaism was more a cultural influence than a religious practice.

When Sidney developed a taste for wearing more stylish clothes than were available in their own store, his obliging parents encouraged him to find apparel in more fashionable shops, wanting him to fit in and make friends among the children of successful families. They were pleased when, in high school, he made friends with a boy whose father owned the largest department store in town. The family had a tennis court and, tennis being his favorite sport next to basketball, Sidney became a regular visitor. The Garfields were rapidly and deliberately becoming middle-class Americans, able — and, usually, willing — to pay for Sidney's more sophisticated lifestyle. When Sidney would grow too extravagant, Isaac would chide him with the nickname "Rockefeller." Other times, his stubbornness earned him another nickname, "Mule."

If Sidney's social skills were progressing nicely, his scholastic record was outstanding. Both in grammar school and at Battin High School he showed great promise, and Bertha and Isaac, like many immigrant parents, wanted a career for their son that would assure social respectability and financial security. While he was still in high school, they chose a career in medicine for him, without consulting him. "Mule," meanwhile, knew he wanted to be an architect or an engineer. Both were natural choices for an ambitious student in an era of great marvels like the Panama Canal, the early skyscrapers, and rapid advances in aircraft design. Sidney already was sketching and modeling some of the great buildings he dreamed of designing.

A collision of wills came when Bertha and Isaac learned the state was giving an examination for scholarships to Rutgers, the State University of New Jersey. They were certain Sidney would pass and could earn a free medical education. As the deadline approached for applying, his parents broke the news that he would be taking the test. Sidney found the idea terrifying. He pleaded with his parents to let him study what he wanted. They refused. He begged! No, they insisted. Decades later, his sister vividly recalled how Sidney burst into tears and sobbed into a handkerchief, "I can't stand the sight of blood!" But his parents left him no choice and he applied to take the scholarship examination.

Even sitting for the examination was an honor. Only 60 students in the entire state qualified and only two passed. One was Sidney Garfield. And so, with great reluctance, he gave up his engineering aspirations. How he handled his regrets hints at a trait that emerged to become a lifelong ability: Make the best out of difficult circumstances. As he said many years later, "Something good comes out of everything." If it was a cliché, it was nonetheless a deeply held, lifelong belief.

✤ Chapter 2 ✤

The Great Depression and "Social Medicine"

At Rutgers, Garfield applied himself to pre-medical studies with energy and enthusiasm. To his surprise, he grew to enjoy them. After his sophomore year, his parents moved to Los Angeles, and to remain near the family, Sidney transferred to the University of Southern California (USC), where he completed his Bachelor of Science degree in 1924. For his medical education, he chose the University of Iowa, which had a top-ranked medical school. It also had a chapter of the historically Jewish Zeta Beta Tau fraternity, which he had joined at Rutgers during his freshman year and which he re-joined at Iowa. Whatever drew him to Iowa, the decision served him well as he formed professional relationships there that were important to him for years to come. When he completed his medical degree in 1928, he was awarded a one-year internship at Chicago's highly regarded Michael Reese Hospital, an institution financed by the fortune of a 19th century Jewish immigrant and committed to serving all Chicago residents regardless of race, creed, or nationality. This commitment to egalitarian service fit well with Garfield's own immigrant background and his maturing values.

Following the Michael Reese internship, Garfield returned to Southern California for a second one-year internship at Los Angeles County General Hospital, where he became interested in a surgical specialty that led him to a three-year residency from 1930 to 1933. During that time, Los Angeles County's new hospital was under construction, a 19-story facility touted as the largest hospital in the world when actress Mary Pickford laid the cornerstone in 1930. Its teaching hospital relationship with the USC School of Medicine was already established and, like Michael Reese, it emerged during the Great Depression as a vital force in extending care to the underserved.

Over the new entrance, its commitment to community service was literally carved in stone: *"Erected by the citizens of the County of Los Angeles to provide hospital care for the acutely ill and suffering to whom the doctors of the attending staff give their services without charge in order that no citizen of the county shall be deprived of health for lack of such care and services."* The progressive architecture of the new county hospital, as health care scholar Laurie Zoloth has observed, seemed part of the dialogue over what "social" medicine could achieve: "… the very architecture [is] a tangible transmitter of the optimistic culture of American life … [of] the deepest aspirational principle behind the construction of the systems of health care."

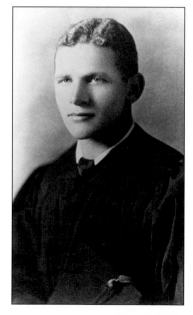

Garfield started his residency at a time when the newly professionalized medical community was in ferment, struggling to find ways to deal with the challenges of a country wracked by the Great Depression, a country becoming so desperate there was even serious talk in some circles of revolution. Health care was just one of the challenges. Unemployment, racial barriers, and rising medical costs kept millions of Americans from proper care. By the end of his residency, 15 million Americans — about one in four — were unemployed, and almost every bank in the country had closed. Franklin D. Roosevelt had been elected President and, within his first 100 days of taking office on March 1, 1933, he had launched scores of New Deal programs to help Americans regain a sense of hope.

Sidney Garfield's graduation portrait, University of Iowa School of Medicine, 1928.

These were dynamic times within the medical community. The national Committee on the Costs of Medical Care, a blue-ribbon group made up of 48 outstanding physi-

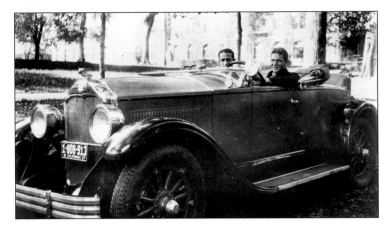

Sidney Garfield at the wheel of a 1927 Buick roadster, probably his first car, purchased about the time he graduated from medical school.

cians, economists, and other health care professionals, was chaired by Ray Lyman Wilbur, M.D., past president of the American Medical Association (AMA), former dean of the Stanford University Medical School, and longtime president of Stanford University. Created at a time when medical costs were soaring and the vast majority of Americans had little or no access to quality medical care, the committee sought ways to make health care more affordable and more available to the average American. Its highly controversial recommendations focused primarily on economic and organizational models for the reform of American medicine — multispecialty group medical practice; a focus on preventing illness as well as caring for the sick; some system, such as prepayment, to more broadly share the burden of cost; and better coordination of hospital facilities to maximize care delivery. This approach was in sharp contrast to the traditionally autonomous, solo practice model of medicine favored by the AMA. Many of the committee's ideas were so noxious to the mainstream medical community that they were soundly rejected. The AMA condemned them as "incitement to revolution," and the *New York Times* dubbed them "socialized medicine." To what extent Garfield was caught up in the ideological controversy, which lasted for more than five years, is unknown, but given his subsequent embrace of many of the ideas promoted by the committee, it is safe to assume that he followed the debate with some interest.

In any case, at Los Angeles County General Hospital the medical issues behind the debate were practical problems to be solved. As at other public hospitals during the Great Depression, physicians had to deal with rapidly growing health care demands from an increasingly desperate and destitute population, at the same time that the science and technology of medicine was expanding exponentially. At Los Angeles

County General Hospital, all of this was occurring in a state-of-the-art facility that was literally rising around them as they attempted to grapple with the challenges.

In this climate, Garfield and his colleagues loved the teaching hospital atmosphere, with its relationship to the medical school at USC, which had just reopened after a seven-year closure. A big part of the hospital's attraction was its commitment to meet the needs of the community in a way that also served the academic needs of the interns and the medical students from USC. This was thanks in large measure to Dr. Phoebus Berman, who had been appointed medical director in 1923. During the years of Garfield's residency, Berman used the association with USC's reopened medical school to help transform the hospital's internship program into something much more like a modern university teaching hospital.

It would be hard to overestimate the influence of Garfield's residency at Los Angeles County General Hospital on his later career and on the founding of Kaiser Permanente. Garfield was clearly immersed in the dynamic world of young physicians learning and working and playing together in an exciting, demanding medical setting. County General interns and residents of the early 1930s lived together in a dormitory building beside the new hospital. Garfield and his roommates, Raymond "Ray" Kay and Justin Wallace "Wally" Neighbor, became lifelong friends.

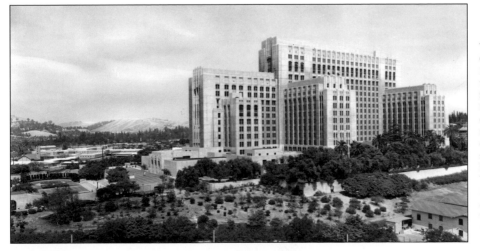

The new Los Angeles County General Hospital was built in the early 1930s when Sidney Garfield was in residence. It was dedicated to providing medical services to all, often without charge, so that no one would be deprived of care. This view is from 1960. Photo credit: Los Angeles Herald Examiner Collection, Los Angeles Public Library.

Inevitably, they all found themselves caught up in the problems of the times. In years to come, Kay and Neighbor would join Garfield as pioneers in group medical practice and in the development of Kaiser Permanente. As Kay later described the impact of the Depression and Los Angeles County General Hospital: "… we were at a point of social change, where the Great Depression and the innovative policies of the Roosevelt Administration began to emphasize the need to help those who could not help themselves. So [our] thinking and actions … were a product of the times."

Garfield was particularly attracted to this highly collegial environment, where everyone learned from everyone else, including, as it happened, two of Garfield's University of Iowa acquaintances, who joined him at County General: Charles Rowan, M.D., who had been Chairman of the Surgery Department in Iowa, and Clarence "C.J." Berne, M.D., a former classmate and gifted young surgeon. The new hospital, in short, was an exciting place because it was full of bright, mostly young, and idealistic physicians grappling together with life and death issues on a daily basis. Internist Ray Kay, in later years, often talked about the importance of his time there with Garfield: "When he was on duty at night as a surgical resident seeing all the acute abdomens and other acute cases, I would very frequently join him, and I learned a tremendous amount. Likewise, he would spend a lot of time with me in my medical wards and we would learn from each other … We shared our patients, and shared our knowledge, and learned a great deal … Whatever the patient needed, we could do for them. Whatever we needed — the lab work, the X-rays, or to diagnose them, or to treat them — we were able to do, and there was nothing that stopped us. That seemed to be wonderful.

"We then started thinking, 'Wouldn't it be wonderful if we could really practice as a doctor with a group of doctors where you could share knowledge, and share experience, and share patients, and where you could take care of people with no economic blocks?'"

What Kay, Garfield, and their County General colleagues were experiencing and dreaming of were the largely unheralded and misunderstood advantages of prepaid, group medical practice — a form of physician organization and cooperation that the AMA still equated with socialism. "We recognized," said Kay, "the importance of being able to provide all necessary medical studies and treatment with no economic barriers. We also appreciated the fact that we were able to develop professionally through sharing patients and learning from the other physicians with whom we worked."

Garfield later made the case for the virtues of group practice to physicians in Portland, Oregon, when he told a meeting of the Multnomah County Medical Association in 1945: "It has always been a paradox that group practice is the method used to teach medicine of the highest type — all university medical schools are group practice operations — yet the individual physician is taught to go into solo practice. Group practice is essential because as medical knowledge increases in mass and complexity, no one doctor can learn the entire field … This produces both quality and economy. Quality, because the doctors participating are specialists, because consultation is easy, and because of the stimulus resulting from working with well-trained [physicians] in various fields. Economy results from the use of common facilities, records, office space, and equipment, and elimination of waste of travel." But perhaps most important was the power this could bring to preventing illness.

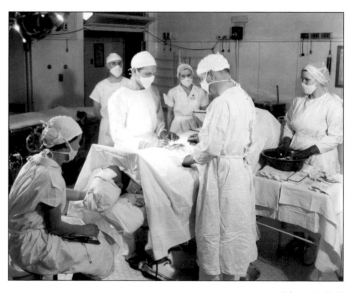

Sidney Garfield performing surgery, probably during his time as the so-called "Super Resident" at Los Angeles County General Hospital.

It was here that Garfield summed things up from a patient point of view in a simple phrase, "The people of this country … don't want to get sick."

It was with some irony, then, that the medical establishment saw Garfield's vision of widespread group medical practice as unethical and socialistic when Garfield saw it as an extension into the community of the university teaching hospital model, bluntly telling the annual meeting of the AMA in Chicago (Appendix 1)

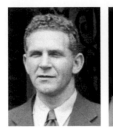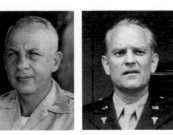

Fellow residents (left to right) Sidney Garfield, Ray Kay, and Wally Neighbor. Said Garfield, "We grew up at the County Hospital."

a year before the Portland speech, "Group practice needs no experimentation. It has proved itself in the clinics and universities of this country."

John G. Smillie, M.D., another group medical practice pioneer who trained at Los Angeles County General Hospital and later wrote a history of The Permanente Medical Group in Northern California, believed that the "socially responsive hospital setting where patients were treated without consideration of payment" was formative in Garfield's development. "Garfield, Kay, and Neighbor shared with each other the fascinating clinical experiences of Los Angeles County General Hospital ... The young physicians absorbed a sense of medicine as a form of social practice that was part and parcel, not only of Los Angeles County, but of America itself during the Depression years. Under the assault of economic hardship, the social dimension of American experience was asserting itself against an already established philosophy of individualism. These young doctors were learning not only from each other and from the teams of physicians at Los Angeles County, but also from the philosophy of social responsibility that animated a great public hospital at a time of economic stress ..."

This was the context in which Garfield declared many years later, when speaking of himself and other founding physicians of Kaiser Permanente, "We grew up at the County Hospital."

It was this extraordinary training and experience that Garfield carried into the Southern California desert in 1933 as he set out to make his way as a newly minted physician in an economic environment every bit as bleak as the scrublands surrounding Desert Center. Here, he experimented with ideas rather than philosophized about them, and his failures and successes forged the ideas that would make him one of the greatest health care innovators of the 20th century.

Chapter 3

Revolution in the Economics of Medicine

Although Garfield's challenges at Contractors General Hospital were many, the hazards and hardships he faced in the desert ultimately were dwarfed by the prospect of financial ruin. When money began to run out, the only thing keeping the hospital open was the fact that his small staff — and only nurse, Betty Runyen — had been working without pay for seven months. Bankruptcy was on the horizon when Garfield was saved by a most unlikely source — two insurance executives. They offered to prepay the cost of medical care for aqueduct workers, a proposal that came in the nick of time.

"Our financial position became rather precarious," recalled Garfield. "Payrolls couldn't be met, creditors were unhappy and becoming unpleasant, and it became evident our hospital would have to close." That prospect, however, was as unwelcome for the aqueduct contractors as it was for Garfield. They had become accustomed to having a hospital nearby to provide medical care for their workers. Enter Alonzo B. "A.B." Ordway and Harold Hatch from San Francisco-based Industrial Indemnity Exchange, the largest insurance company on the Colorado River Aqueduct project. Ordway, a former construction supervisor, was executive vice president. Hatch, a brilliant engineer partially crippled by a spinal deformity, was the chief planner and strategist.

Different aspects of their work brought Ordway and Hatch through Desert

Center periodically, and Contractors General had become a friendly oasis from the desert. It was air conditioned, attractive, and comfortable, with the added bonus of the charming and strikingly attractive nurse Runyen, who was a terrific hostess. The two men visited regularly and became good friends with Garfield, despite Ordway's opinion that Garfield was spending too much money equipping what was only a temporary hospital. Garfield, in turn, argued that he "couldn't work without decent equipment."

Hatch saw that he would have his own financial problems if Contractors General went bankrupt. As an insurance underwriter, he needed to control costs; as the representative of big employers who needed medical care for their workers, he depended on Contractors General to provide local medical care rather than having to transport

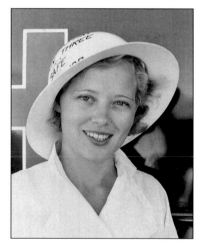

Betty Runyen, Sidney Garfield's nurse at Contractors General Hospital, sporting a hard hat awarded to aqueduct workers for "a safe and clean job," July 1934.

all cases to Los Angeles. So on one of his visits, he made a proposal: "Why don't you make an arrangement with our insurance company whereby we pay you a certain percent of our insurance premiums and then we won't have to fuss around about bills and so forth?" He was talking about prepayment — a predetermined, prepaid premium per worker to cover certain medical services. At the time, Industrial Indemnity was allocating 25 percent of its workers' compensation premium to medical and hospital expenses. Hatch said he would be willing to give half of that to Garfield to care for workers' job-related injuries. It amounted to a nickel a day per worker in Depression-era dollars. Garfield accepted. "I did a little arithmetic and it seemed like more money than we were making anyway … We had nothing to lose."

Garfield's cash flow improved immediately. With a guaranteed weekly income, expenses could be budgeted and the payroll could be met. Creditors soon were paid off. Most important, he recalled, "We were able to provide these workers with all the medical and hospital care they needed for industrial accidents."

Then, in a moment of entrepreneurial inspiration, Garfield realized he could expand prepayment to cover the total health of the workers, both on the job and off the job. After all, he already had the hospital and medical equipment in place. He figured that if the men paid another nickel a day out of their own pockets, he could offer them *comprehensive* medical care. They could have the kind of care only the wealthiest of Americans could pay for in that era for about the price of a soda or cup of coffee. Garfield presented the idea to the contractors, who eagerly sold it to their workers. About 95 percent of the workforce signed up.

With Garfield's revenue stream essentially doubled, he built two more hospitals. One was at Parker Dam on the Colorado River, at the eastern end of the aqueduct. The other, part of another massive federal water project designed to bring irrigation water to the Imperial Valley, was about 130 miles further down

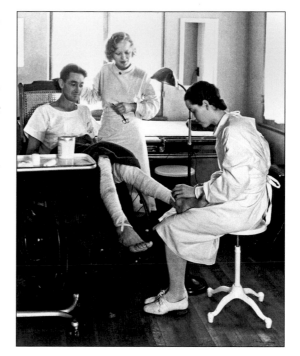

Nurse Betty Runyen with student nurse Pat Allen with an unidentified burn victim at Contractors General Hospital.

the Colorado River at Imperial Dam, near Yuma, Arizona. To make care more accessible to the construction workers, Garfield built and staffed well-equipped first aid stations between the hospitals. His medical practice now stretched across 150 miles of desert and, he said, "We had no more trouble trying to collect bills. The workers had no more concern about paying for their medical care and … [we] were able to expand our services tremendously."

Ordway and Hatch were equally happy. Prepayment, in Ordway's words, "tied down the insurance company costs to a known amount. The arrangement … worked out very satisfactorily, so much so that it aided us a great deal in getting new insurance business." That success on the insurance side would play out in the future with Ordway's boss, the industrialist Henry J. Kaiser, who owned one-third of Industrial Indemnity. It would be a few more years, however, before Garfield would meet "The Boss" and begin a personal and business relationship that would reshape both of their lives and help to transform American health care.

In the meantime, Garfield realized it was the healthy, dues-paying members who were the source of his hospital's income, rather than the sick and injured patients he'd been relying on. It was natural, even inevitable, that he would add one more critical element to his evolving system of medical care — accident prevention. This innovation had a three-fold impact: fewer lost workdays, reduced workplace injuries, and, because of the reduced demand for services, more money to spend on service improvements. Thus, while Garfield invented neither prepayment nor prevention, he figured out how to combine them to produce the maximum benefit. This visionary ability of Garfield to assemble separate concepts into improved

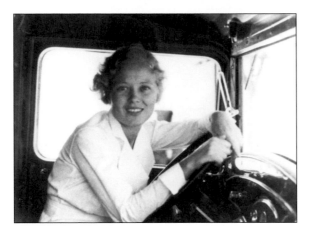

Nurse Betty Runyen at the wheel of a 1932 Ford ambulance at Contractors General Hospital.

approaches to delivering medical care first manifested itself at Desert Center, but he would demonstrate it again and again over coming decades in what he described as his "lesson-by-lesson journey into medical care." As his friend from his residency days, Wally Neighbor, once said, Garfield was "capable of seeing opportunities for achievement where the average person sees none."

The combination of prepayment and prevention paid great dividends for all concerned at Contractors General. "We had been anxious to have sick men or injured men come into the hospital because that meant income and we could continue to exist," Garfield explained. "It was embarrassing to me to want people to get hurt." Prepayment meant he would be better off financially if there were fewer injuries to treat. By reducing demand for care, there would be more money available to hire staff, buy better medical equipment, build new hospitals and first aid clinics, and keep the premiums low. Rather than sitting around waiting for people to get hurt to make a living, he now began to look creatively at how to reduce injuries. His prevention work began in earnest. "We started to do safety engineering … We would get a bunch of nail punctures from a job and we would go out there and get them to clean up the nails. Or we would get a lot of head injuries … and we would get them to shore up the tunnels better."

In short, Garfield reversed the traditional economics of medicine, in which physicians are paid only when a patient is ill. Instead, Garfield would benefit by keeping his patients healthy and accident-free. It was a lesson he would remind himself of in later years with a newspaper clipping he kept in his desk drawer describing the tradition in ancient China, where a physician was paid only while his patient was healthy, not while his patient was ill.

Prepayment and prevention were the great new ideas that sprang up and flourished in the hostile desert environment, and they helped Garfield look at medical care in ways that few practicing physicians had dared. But as exciting as they were, he still dreamed of the great new idea he had taken away from County General — the possibilities of group practice. Here in the desert, though, his medical practice was spread over 150 miles of sparsely populated scrublands. It was not conducive to creating a group medical practice or putting all care under one roof. So Garfield dreamed of returning to Los Angeles to set up a

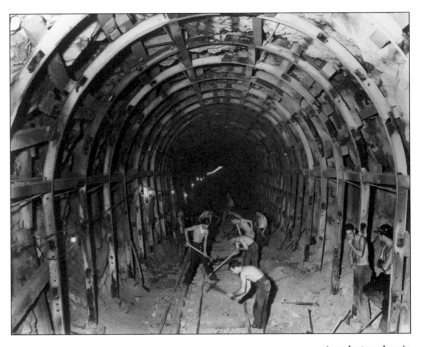

Aqueduct workers in one of the giant tunnels constructed near Garfield's Contractors General Hospital.

group medical practice when the aqueduct work came to an end, as it was soon scheduled to do. Before that could happen, though, fate would intervene in the persons of Edgar F. Kaiser and his father, Henry J.

❦ Chapter 4 ❦

A Fateful House Call

After five years in the desert, Sidney Garfield had a chain of three Contractors General Hospitals, first aid stations, and money in the bank. In 1938, with aqueduct construction nearing an end, he was thinking about his future, including the tempting possibilities for private practice in Los Angeles. Time, however, still was too short for deep contemplation. Garfield was the only surgeon serving the three hospitals, and his life on the desert remained hectic. Driving from hospital to clinic to hospital in his two-door Buick convertible roadster, he would sometimes arrive at one of his hospitals before dawn and nap on the operating room table. In the morning, he would wake up, scrub, and start surgery.

To avoid losing valuable time racing back and forth across the desert, he arranged to have telephone messages left for him along his route at gas stations where he could make a quick stop to find out if he was needed at a particular hospital or clinic. He called it his "pony express route." One day when he stopped, a message awaited him from A.B. Ordway at Industrial Indemnity asking him to telephone as soon as possible. That call would alter the course of his life.

"Sidney," Ordway said, "Edgar Kaiser, Henry's son, is in charge of building the Grand Coulee Dam on the Columbia River. He's asked me to help him locate someone to take over medical care for the workers on the dam. I nominated you for the job. Will you go up to Portland and talk to him about it?"

"No," Garfield said. He explained he had had his fill of remote industrial work camps.

"Well, he wants you to come up and see him."

"Not a chance, Mr. Ordway. I want to get into something permanent. I'm planning on going into practice in Los Angeles."

Ordway begged him to fly to Portland as a personal favor. Garfield finally agreed, but only out of friendship with Ordway, whose suggestion of prepayment had saved him from bankruptcy. However, he insisted he only would offer Edgar advice about how to set up a medical care program. Under no circumstances would he take a job in the eastern Washington desert, some 400 miles up the Columbia River from Portland.

It was a long trip to Portland, a lumbering, uncomfortable five-hour flight from Los Angeles. When Garfield arrived, he was in no mood to be kept waiting. But that's what he was asked to do when he showed up at the posh Multnomah Hotel, "the grand lady of Fourth Avenue," in downtown Portland. It was there that Edgar Kaiser maintained a temporary office. When Garfield called Kaiser's office from the lobby, the secretary said she would call him when Kaiser was ready to see him. No doubt irritated, Garfield checked into a room and sat by the telephone. Around noon, and no call from Kaiser's secretary, Garfield telephoned her again. Kaiser was still too busy to see him.

By mid-afternoon, Garfield was angry. He phoned the Portland airport. The only flight back to Los Angeles was late that evening. Fuming as the afternoon turned to evening, he began rehearsing a speech to preemptively turn Kaiser down: "Mr. Kaiser, I'm not interested in this job. Thank you. Good-bye." Finally, around six o'clock, the telephone rang. Edgar Kaiser finally was ready to see him. Garfield walked up one flight of stairs to Kaiser's suite, hoping their business could be completed as quickly as possible so he could head home.

Garfield knocked on the door, and was surprised to be greeted by a young woman known for her alluring charm. Sue Kaiser, Edgar's wife, wore a warm smile, and she was clearly relieved to see a physician at her door. "Dr. Garfield," she said, "It's so nice of you to come. I'm so happy you're here." She explained she thought her daughter, Becky, might have the measles. Garfield, caught off guard, put aside the little speech he had prepared. He set about examining young Becky, who indeed did have the measles. Garfield's anger was defused. "When I went to see Edgar, I wasn't as mad as I had been."

Kaiser, however, was no more predisposed to working with Garfield than Garfield was to working with Kaiser. After meeting Garfield for only a few minutes, Kaiser decided he didn't like him. That was not surprising. First impressions of

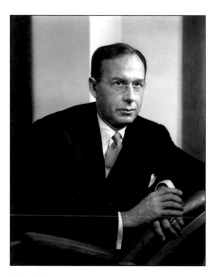

Edgar Kaiser, son of Henry J., oversaw construction of the Grand Coulee Dam on the Columbia River.

the shy, dapperly dressed Garfield in those days were often unremarkable, if not downright negative. As one writer who knew him well said, "Garfield was a man whom you'd not pick out of the human mass as a leader." Kaiser wasted no time telephoning Ordway in San Francisco.

"Ord, for God's sake, who did you send me?" Kaiser barked.

Ordway was frustrated. He knew the real Garfield and knew that he was the physician for the job. He reminded Kaiser that he had warned him his first impression might not be a good one. He again urged him to spend a few days with Garfield, not a few minutes. "Edgar," Ordway said, "I told you not to make a decision until you had talked to this man a long time." Relenting, Kaiser took Ordway's advice. He managed to persuade Garfield to stay the night and have a look at the hospital in Mason City the following day. During their six-hour drive, the two men, very different in background and experience but close in age, began to warm to each other.

The 30-year-old Kaiser asked the young doctor about his work in the Mojave Desert, and Garfield, 32, explained how it was organized around prepayment and injury prevention. Kaiser explained his problem at Coulee. The Kaiser Company led a consortium of contractors — Consolidated Builders — that had lost out on their bid to build the so-called low dam that would be the foundation for the final Coulee Dam. Now, they had won the bid for the "high dam" that would raise the water level 350 feet above the Columbia River's bed. They had inherited the Mason City Hospital, which had been built by the earlier contractors to serve dam construction workers. However, the 75-bed hospital already was in disrepair and was poorly run with a two-tiered system of care that the unionized workers had grown to hate. After their members' bad experience with the original contractors, union leaders were adamant that they, not Kaiser, should run any medical care program at the dam.

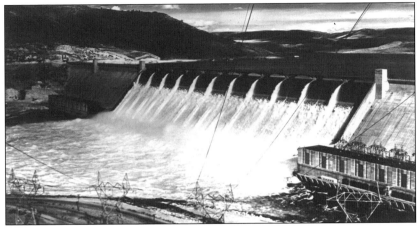

Grand Coulee Dam on the Columbia River, the largest man-made structure in history at the time.

But Edgar Kaiser believed it was important for the employers to provide the care. He was committed to the idea that both workers and managers deserved high-quality medical care in a single system. He and his father had dealt with medical care inequities on construction projects before — while building a highway across Cuba and at the Hoover and Bonneville Dams. They had grown frustrated with traditional industrial practices. Garfield listened and was impressed with Kaiser's social consciousness, and how the construction manager seemed to understand Garfield's ideas about injury prevention and prepayment. Mason City at last appeared in the distance. Through the windshield Garfield saw something that suddenly sold him on the idea of starting a medical care program for the Kaisers.

The Mason City site that Garfield saw as the car descended into the valley was remarkable. Compared with the temporary aqueduct work camps scattered across more than 150 miles of Mojave Desert, the new town of Mason City had been built on a flat plot of land on the east side of the Columbia River just below the dam site. Designed to be the world's first "all-electric city," the goal was to demonstrate the convenience of electricity and to promote its use to secure a firm market for the power that would be generated when the dam was finished. The town cost more than a million Depression-era dollars to build. There were more than 300 houses, several dormitories, a 1,000-seat cookhouse, and the Mason City Hospital, all for thousands of dam workers and their dependents who were moving into the area. "Instead of being spread across the desert," said Garfield, "the work at Coulee was all at one location. Here was the opportunity to get a group practice of specialists together in one location as we had dreamed about in the desert, with everything we needed for good care under one roof. I took the job."

Though only a few years old, the Mason City Hospital was in serious disrepair. Paint was peeling from the exterior walls. There was no landscaping. Its poor reputation made it hard to recruit doctors. Edgar Kaiser told Garfield to

Garfield had to totally renovate the old hospital at the Grand Coulee construction headquarters in Mason City to accommodate the thousands of workers living on site.

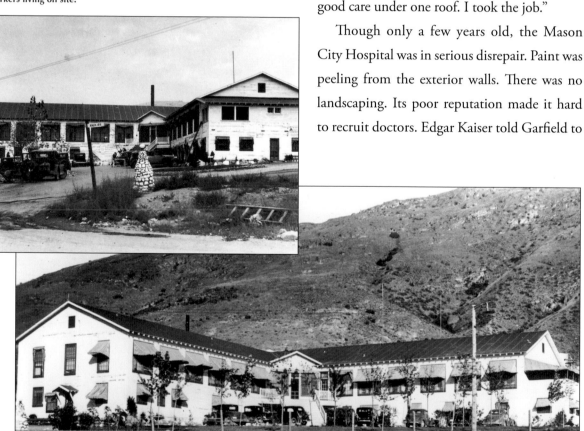

fix it up in whatever manner he wanted, which he did. He had it painted inside and out. Workmen repaired doors and windows, hung curtains, re-outfitted three operating rooms, and bought the most modern medical equipment. Only Garfield's request for air conditioning was rejected as a "luxury," which put Garfield in a bind. He already had promised it to the labor leaders. So he paid for it out of his own pocket from money he had saved from the aqueduct project, and even hauled the used air conditioning equipment from his original Contractors General Hospital up to Mason City. For his new air conditioning equipment, Garfield negotiated a good discount from a Spokane company. In the end, Edgar Kaiser reimbursed him for the equipment and took the heat of complaints from some of his profit-minded business colleagues. He responded by pointedly reminding them they were not providing health care to make money. As manager of the dam project and son of Henry J., he told them he would be satisfied if the medical care program simply broke even.

❧ Chapter 5 ❧

The Final Dress Rehearsal

Beginning in 1938, Garfield threw himself into the work of creating the more complex medical delivery system that he dreamed about in the Mojave Desert. Over the next few years, he would experiment with connecting ideas about prevention and prepaid financing with group medical practice and facilities all under a single roof.

The first task — recruiting well-trained physicians willing to move to the remote site of "the Grand Coulee" — was a major challenge. He turned to where he had the most contacts, urban Southern California, but with little success. Even in the Depression, few qualified specialists were anxious to move to such a desolate place.

His one early recruiting success was of his old friend from Los Angeles County General Hospital, Wally Neighbor, who was a Washington state native. While Garfield was at Desert Center, Neighbor had become physician-in-residence at the luxurious Arrowhead Springs Hotel, a resort in the San Bernardino Mountains about 125 miles west of Garfield's little hospital. It was a Southern California playground frequented by Hollywood stars of the 1930s, including luminaries like Mary Pickford, Spencer Tracy, and Humphrey Bogart. During those years, Garfield frequently visited Neighbor at the hotel for rest and relaxation. It was there that Garfield met and dated for a time the lovely film star Alice Faye. "It wasn't as if he went out into the desert and became a monk," Neighbor once quipped.

Perhaps, with their connections in the Hollywood crowd, the two young physicians were perfectly poised to become some of the original "Beverly Hills doctors." However, that would never come to pass even if they did fantasize about it. Neighbor paid a visit to Coulee and jumped at the chance to join Garfield. Although he had had experiences at Arrowhead Springs that he "wouldn't trade for anything," Neighbor, tired of seeing movie colony neurotics, had lost any desire to continue working with Hollywood stars. "It was not the most exciting kind of medical care," he recalled. Garfield was thrilled. He named Neighbor chief of staff in Mason City.

In reminiscing about his first trip to Coulee, Neighbor recalled an episode that endeared Garfield to him and sheds light on the loyalty Garfield earned from the people he hired. "There was no hotel then and Sid showed me a bed and said, 'You can stay here for the night and there is a room over here that I'll stay in.'" When Neighbor awoke in the morning and stuck his head into Garfield's room, Garfield already was up and gone. And there was no bed, only a set of box springs on the floor with a blanket over it. "He had slept there and let me have the bed," Neighbor said. "I think that tells a lot about Sid … He's unselfish and he would go to all ends to make people happy."

The trait served Garfield well. It helped him create a team he could lead and inspire even during his extended absences — for Garfield wanted to split his time between Coulee and Los Angeles, where he had been offered an appointment to become the first supervising resident in surgery for the USC Surgery Service. The offer was extended by Dr. Clarence Berne, a classmate in medical school who by then was chairman of the Department of Surgery at USC. Neighbor, Garfield theorized, would be a strong chief of staff. Once the Mason City Hospital was up and running smoothly, Garfield could then spend a good chunk of time in Los Angeles teaching at County General Hospital.

Before he could take on the teaching assignment, however, Garfield first had to recruit more physicians and nurses. Initially, he thought he could count on Neighbor's Washington connections and the fact that he was offering physicians monthly salaries of $500 to $600 — double those of most fee-for-service physicians in the Northwest. Then he learned just how bad the reputation was that plagued the medical care at

Mason City. County hospital residents in both Seattle and Portland turned him down cold; as did everyone else he approached.

Garfield next looked to San Francisco County Hospital, where he managed to interest Ray Gillette, a Stanford Medical School-trained obstetrician and gynecologist who, like Neighbor, was a Washington native. Gillette not only accepted, he recommended a friend, a promising 27-year-old San Francisco County Hospital surgical resident, also from Stanford, Cecil C. Cutting.

Garfield telephoned Cutting and described the prepaid industrial care program he was setting up. He offered Cutting the position of chief surgeon. Cutting agreed to think about it. However, a few days later Cutting telephoned Garfield. Could he come to Stanford? Cutting wanted to meet in person, and he wanted Garfield to explain his idea about assembling prepayment, prevention, and group medical practice into a system of care to Cutting's mentor, Stanford Medical School Dean Loren Chandler. Cutting wanted to hear Dr. Chandler's views before committing himself. The meeting was disastrous. Chandler was wedded to the status quo and saw Garfield as a medical revolutionary to be avoided. It was a preview of what Garfield could expect in the future from fee-for-service medicine and its view of prepaid group practice as "medical socialism."

Chandler declared Garfield's program "unethical" because, he believed, physicians would be employed by the contractors and, by working for non-physicians, would violate the AMA's Canon of Ethics. He told Cutting he would have a professional black mark against him for the rest of his life if he went to work for Garfield. He might even be barred from the AMA. Garfield protested. He explained that he was a member of the AMA and that the physicians worked for him — not the Kaisers. Chandler was adamant. He could never agree to Cutting going to Grand Coulee. Garfield was facing more resistance than he expected.

Cutting asked for a few days to think things over. Like Neighbor, he was attracted by the potential experience Mason City offered a young physician. "To go as chief surgeon to a new hospital ... would give me a lot more experience the first few years," he reasoned. "I was young, eager, active, [and] anxious to work, so I called

Dr. Garfield and told him … I'd go up and take a look." When Cutting arrived at Coulee, Neighbor, as chief of staff, was at work helping with the remodeling and minor additions to the hospital. Neighbor and Garfield showed Cutting around. They described their plans. Their competence, honesty, and enthusiasm overcame any doubts Cutting had left. He signed on.

Garfield's recruiting efforts gradually turned a corner. Soon, the medical team that he assembled was a tapestry of friendships and personal relationships that flourished in the Washington wilderness. Neighbor and Garfield already were longtime friends. Cutting, Gillette, and Richard Moore, another Stanford-trained resident, in surgery and orthopedics, all came from San Francisco County Hospital. Charles Olson, an internist with an interest in endocrinology who knew the three of them from Stanford, also joined the group, as did Eugene Wiley, a general surgeon who was a medical school classmate of Garfield.

It was like old home week for some of the nurses, support staff, and physician wives as well. Pete Bashta, the hospital's orderly and ambulance driver, along with his wife, Yvonne, the housekeeper, followed Garfield from one of his Contractors General Hospital sites. They worked under Rex Hamby, administrator of the third of Garfield's desert hospitals, who now was administrator at Mason City. As time went on, the interrelationships grew more numerous. Hamby's assistant, Frank Stewart, met and married his wife, Alta, a nurse at Coulee; Dr. Olson, also married a nurse, Evelyn Sanger. Three physician wives who also were nurses — Millie Cutting, Ysabel Moore and Hazel Gillette — had known each other since their nursing school days at Stanford. The San Francisco doctors recruited four nurses with whom they had worked at San Francisco County, including Winnie Wetherill, who later married Wally Neighbor.

The work was hard over the next few years while the dam went up. But there was a family-like bond among the young medical staff of Sidney R. Garfield and Associates. The Cuttings' home, a converted schoolhouse, became the center of social activity and parties would float from one home to another. "Being all together in quite a social group, all liking each other … we really didn't feel too cut off," Garfield recalled of that time. "We felt like we were really enjoying ourselves." Garfield, of course, was less cut off than the others because he traveled back and forth, administering his program from afar whenever his teaching duties took him to Los Angeles County General Hospital, where he had taken that "super resident" job, as it became known. His growing experience at managing from a distance would serve him well during World War II.

Under Garfield's leadership, this group of men and women, physicians and nurses, built a fundamentally new system of care for 15,000 workers and their dependents. It included a small multispecialty group medical practice; clinical and hospital facilities under one roof; a focus on the prevention of illness and injury; virtually all financed through prepayment. The pieces of Garfield's dream were falling into place. The new health care system even included the wives and children of the men building the dam, an expansion of care for which Garfield had to guess at a prepaid premium since there was nothing comparable on which to estimate expenses. He finally settled on 50 cents a month for adult dependents and 25 cents for a child. Like the hospital air conditioning, Garfield created the family plan at the behest of the unions, but this time with backing from Edgar Kaiser.

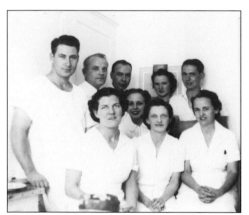

Cecil Cutting, center, back row, with his surgery department staff at Mason City Hospital in 1940. Millie Cunningham, the nurse center of front row, later married Dr. Cutting and became a prominent figure in Kaiser Permanente history during World War II.

And, said Garfield, stepping into this world of the unknown proved to be "the most impressive lesson of our experience." Suddenly, prepayment and prevention revealed their ultimate power. Paid and freed to work on keeping people well, the young medical team found it could improve people's health and keep costs from skyrocketing. With health care at a price people could afford, the workers and their wives and children began coming in to see the doctor sooner, enabling early diagnosis and treatment to further head off serious illness.

"Prior to this family plan, when walking through the corridors of our little hospital at Coulee, we would see very sick women and children," Garfield recalled. "After the plan had been in operation for three or four months, there was a noticeable change in the severity level of illness ... The reason was simple. These people, with the barrier of cost for medical service removed, were coming to us early in their illnesses ... Ruptured appendices changed to simple appendices; terminal pneumonias became early pneumonias. Certain medical conditions disappeared entirely, (such as) diphtheria and mastoidectomies."

Suddenly, too, community residents who were not even part of the Kaiser operations showed up for care — willing to pay for it out of pocket. "We began to realize what was happening," said Garfield. "This large group of women and children who had been receiving very little medical care and who had been staying away from our hospital until seriously ill were now coming to us early and frequently. They were talking about their experience over the back fence, in the grocery store, wherever they met other people. This discussion of medical matters stimulated the medical consciousness of the community ..."

There had been no plan for all of this. Instead, one experiment followed another. If something worked, it was incorporated. If it didn't, it was dropped. Themes began to emerge. Edgar Kaiser had made it clear the medical care program was not to be a profit center within Kaiser industrial enterprises. Putting together group medical practice, services under one roof, and family coverage and joining them to the concepts of prepayment and prevention proved to be a felicitous, if not a deliberately designed, success.

Edgar Kaiser had brought Garfield into the Kaiser enterprises, and when the physician and Henry Kaiser met for the first time, the elder Kaiser immediately understood how all this could benefit people's health. "Young man," Kaiser said, "if your idea is half as good as you say it is ... it's good for the entire country ... Your particular job must be to make sure your model is the very best ..." Together, Garfield and the Kaisers had laid the foundation for what would become Kaiser Permanente. The

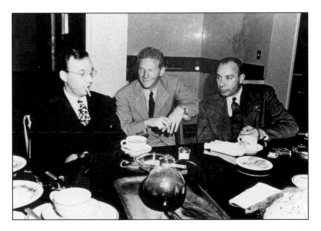

As the Grand Coulee project wound down in 1940, Edgar Kaiser, left, Sidney Garfield, center, and Cecil Cutting reflected on their accomplishments.

Grand Coulee Dam project, Garfield said, was "the final dress rehearsal." When the Japanese bombed Pearl Harbor in 1941, Garfield would be tossed into the toughest laboratory of all, and he would see his ideas play on the world stage, rather than in remote desert landscapes.

❧ Chapter 6 ❧

FDR to Garfield:
"You're *Not* in the Army Now!"

The years at Grand Coulee laid the foundations for the prepaid group practice model of health care for which Garfield would later be known. However, when the job was winding down, he had no idea what the future held. Indeed, as the storm clouds of World War II gathered, Garfield was back at the USC medical school as the "super resident." He had a growing image as a handsome, young, and increasingly successful surgeon. His mentor, Dr. Clarence Berne, was developing his own image as the striking and erudite chairman of the department of surgery. Rumor had it he was the model for "young doctor Kildare" in the Lew Ayers and Lionel Barrymore movies of the late 1930s and early 1940s.

These were heady days for Garfield. He began investing his earnings in Southern California real estate with valued advice from his father. The bachelor doctor now drove a Cadillac. He ate at fine restaurants, including the then-new Earl Carroll Theatre on Sunset Boulevard in the heart of Hollywood, where stars flocked to see spectacular chorus lines on stage for as many as 1,000 diners at once. Garfield clearly appreciated the place. The bumper sticker on his car bore the same slogan as that emblazoned in neon over the entrance to the club: "Through these portals pass the most beautiful girls in the world."

The debonair doctor, often described as having a movie star quality, fit right in. As the famous science writer Paul de Kruif, who came to know him well, later wrote: "He was definitely a young man of mystery. His finely tailored clothes remained unwrinkled because of the economy and careful precision of the way he moved about. He seemed not medical and even a bit Hollywoodish in his elegance, but beneath that he was wiry and gave one the feeling that one had better not get funny with him. His face had high cheekbones and was chiseled in clean lines, photogenic. His hair, cut close, was curly reddish-gold and he was deeply tanned. His gray-green eyes told little because they were usually peering through narrow slits, especially when he smiled, which was often, and yet he seemed to be a sad young man and in repose round his mouth there were deep lines that had been made, I guessed, by some kind of pain, not physical."

At the county hospital, too, Garfield exuded this "star" quality. Sally Bolotin worked for the medical director, Dr. Phoebus Berman, handling the rotations of interns and residents. She watched them react to the "super resident." "I remember he drove a Cadillac and all of the interns and residents were very impressed with him," she recalled. "And apparently he was an excellent teacher because … he would be walking down the hall in his surgical gown and, just like a Pied Piper, all the little interns and residents would follow him down the hall, waiting for a pearl of wisdom to drop." Many decades later, Bolotin recalled both Berman and Garfield as "the two most brilliant men I have ever met."

Heading into the 1940s, Garfield must have imagined unlimited possibilities for himself. Then, Japan bombed Pearl Harbor. The next day, stunned Americans tuned their radios to hear President Franklin D. Roosevelt's voice crackling over the airwaves as he addressed an emergency joint session of Congress: "I ask that the Congress declare that since the unprovoked and dastardly attack by Japan on Sunday, December 7th, 1941, a state of war has existed between the United States and the Japanese empire."

By the tens of thousands, "the greatest generation" began signing up to fight on the front lines or, if not qualified to serve, for the huge Home Front workforce needed to turn out the ships, airplanes, tanks, rifles, boots, and much more to support the American fighting force. Sidney Garfield was among them, immediately enlisting with the 73rd Evacuation Hospital organized by USC's volunteer clinical faculty. First Lieutenant Garfield, who because of an allergy to wool was outfitted at his own cost in a custom-tailored Army uniform, reported to his mentor, Dr. Berne — now Colonel Berne. They prepared to ship out for Burma.

Meanwhile, on the eastern shore of San Francisco Bay, in the sleepy little town of Richmond, Clay Bedford, who had worked for his old friend Edgar Kaiser as chief engineer on the Grand Coulee Dam, was running a new shipyard built by Henry Kaiser. The Kaiser Company had a head start on the American Home Front war, having begun building ships for the British before the attack on Pearl Harbor. The Permanente Metals Corporation, the business entity that ran the Kaiser Shipyards, would quickly expand to four yards and employ almost 100,000 workers, turning Richmond — just a dozen miles north of Kaiser's headquarters in Oakland — into an overnight boomtown. Edgar Kaiser was mounting an identical effort on the Columbia River at Vancouver, Washington, and then across the river in Portland, Oregon. In Fontana — a Southern California desert community 45 miles east of Los Angeles — Henry Kaiser was building his own mill to produce steel for the ships.

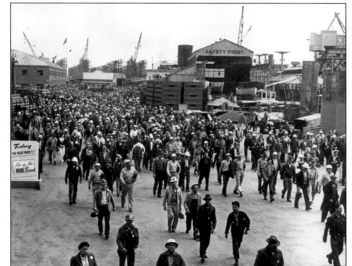

Home Front shipbuilders during a shift change in the Richmond Kaiser Shipyards, now one of the sites of the Rosie the Riveter / World War II Home Front National Historical Park.

Among the early shipbuilders in both Richmond and Vancouver were workers who came from the Coulee job, along with heavy equipment that was moved from Coulee and adapted for shipbuilding. As a Kaiser executive once described the company's wartime shipbuilding attitude: "A ship was nothing but a dam that wouldn't stay put." By the end of World War II, the Kaiser yards and workers — at one point launching a ship every day — set records for shipbuilding never reached before or since.

The explosion of production activity presented enormous challenges. Thousands of people poured into Richmond for the new shipyard jobs, creating shortages of all kinds — housing, schools, and medical care among them. Building 10,000-ton ships was dangerous work. It involved huge machines, heavy lifting, explosive materials, and lots of welding equipment. Civilian injuries — far exceeding those of the military — were numerous despite a heavy emphasis on safety. Scarce medical resources in the community could not handle the amount of medical care needed. Besides, the national shortage of doctors was growing as physicians left their practices for military service. Bedford immediately thought of Garfield and the job he had done at Coulee. He put in a telephone call shortly after Pearl Harbor.

Reached as he was preparing to ship out, Garfield told Bedford he could not help. He was already in the Army. He would head for Burma in a month. Bedford pleaded: "Well, you've got a month. Can you come up and advise me what to do?" In early January of 1942, Garfield, in uniform, traveled north and began conferring with Bedford and Kaiser's other son, Henry Jr., along with his old friends from the Southern California desert, Harold Hatch and A.B. Ordway of Industrial Indemnity. He and Ordway talked almost daily until one day Ordway vanished. No one would tell Garfield where he had gone.

It became clear that delivering medical care to tens of thousands of people in the shipyards would be an unprecedented challenge. The Kaiser team agreed that only Sidney Garfield had the skills and proven experience to tackle it. With that in mind, Ordway had hurried off to Washington, D.C. He carried a special request from Henry Kaiser to President Roosevelt, who granted it. Ordway rushed back to hand Garfield a letter from the Commander in Chief releasing Garfield from the Army because he was needed to provide medical care for the workers who would help carry on the production war on the Home Front.

Garfield was flabbergasted, and somewhat miffed at Ordway: "He hadn't even asked me …" What upset Garfield most was that he did not want to be seen as disloyal by his fellow physicians in the 73rd Evacuation Hospital. He telephoned Colonel Berne to talk it over, but Berne encouraged Garfield to stick with Kaiser. "He thought I could be doing something more important," Garfield said. Berne was right. Garfield, now 35, was about to create the largest civilian medical care program of World War II. It would evolve after the war into the largest not-for-profit private health care delivery system in the world.

Garfield's pace was feverish. The rolls of potential patients grew by hundreds, then thousands, and then tens of thousands as cars, buses, and trains filled with workers headed to the West Coast for Kaiser steel mill and shipyard jobs. In addition to doctors, nurses, pharmacists, laboratory technicians, and ambulance drivers, among others, Garfield needed first aid stations, emergency rooms and four hospitals — a field hospital for emergencies in Richmond, along with three full hospitals, one in Oakland, one in Vancouver, and one at the steel mill in Fontana.

This gigantic endeavor resembled neither the Eastern Washington nor the Southern California desert projects. Coulee was one small hospital by comparison, serving a fraction of the number of patients. Contractors General and its satellite sites were spread over a mere 150 miles compared with the Home Front medical care project that stretched across three major sites from Fontana in Southern California to Vancouver, 1,000 miles to the north on the Washington-Oregon border. Garfield, headquartered at his Oakland hospital, was so busy — and on the road so much — that his administrative assistant Sally Bolotin reported he never even found time to claim an office or even a desk of his own until the end of the war. When he was in town, he mostly would share her desk.

From a medical standpoint, the first workers who arrived in the shipyards were men who were too old, too young, or medically unfit for military service. Garfield jokingly referred to the bulk of these patients as "a walking pathological museum" adding, however, that "in spite of all that, they really built ships, and built them fast."

Next to join the ranks of shipyard laborers were women. The first woman ever to work in an American shipyard was hired by Edgar Kaiser in Vancouver, and soon there were thousands of women in the shipyards. As with women across the Home Front, they became known by the nickname that would stick forever — "Rosie the Riveter," or the "Rosies." Men and women were joined by African-American workers — including women — as racial barriers fell. Chinese workers also joined the team. Soon the shipyards were a multicultural force unparalleled on such a scale. Adding to the racial, ethnic, and gender mix were workers with disabilities — the hearing impaired, men missing limbs and people with other physical handicaps. Today, these civilian war heroes are celebrated at the Rosie the Riveter / World War II Home Front National Historical Park in Richmond and at historic sites including the former Kaiser Shipyards and Garfield's First Aid Station and Richmond Field Hospital. These two sites took in injured workers for emergency care, whereas those needing longer-term hospitalization were taken to his headquarters at the Permanente Foundation Hospital, which had rapidly been constructed out of the ashes and burned-out shell of an abandoned hospital in Oakland.

Among women joining the medical care program staff, Sally Bolotin came to Oakland from Los Angeles County General Hospital. Wanting to help out on the Home Front, she wrote to Garfield asking if she could "come up and help if you have something available." Recalling the frantic days following her arrival in Oakland, she said Garfield put her to work as a "jack of all trades." From her vantage point, gleaned through interviews and letters, comes a rare first-person description of Garfield on the Home Front.

In letters to colleagues, she described the frenetic pace at which new additions were added to the Oakland hospital to keep up with exploding numbers of patients. Because of this constant construction through the war years, Bolotin said the hospital quickly was nicknamed the "Winchester House," a reference to the famous "Winchester Mystery House" in nearby San Jose, to which the eccentric Winchester rifle millionairess, Sarah Winchester, kept adding rooms throughout her life.

Staffing the hospital was reminiscent of Coulee on a larger scale. Just as Garfield had recruited heavily from San Francisco County Hospital for his Mason City Hospital, he now drew heavily from Los Angeles County General Hospital. Bolotin began to recognize more and more faces of her former charges when they were medical residents in Los Angeles. Soon Oakland took on a second nickname — "Los Angeles County Hospital Annex." Notable among these young physicians in mid-1942 was a young doctor named Morris F. Collen, whose asthma had barred him from military duty. He would become one of Garfield's closest colleagues and famous in his own right in postwar American medicine. Also joining Sidney Garfield and Associates, his corporate name, were physicians and nurses from the Coulee days, including Cecil Cutting who came down from Spokane, where he had gone into practice at the Mason Clinic when Grand Coulee Dam was completed.

Bolotin's descriptions of Garfield in letters and in an oral history about the era offer rare insights into the man. Garfield was undergoing a transformation — from a talented and gentlemanly surgeon to creator of a social medicine program that California historian Kevin Starr would describe six decades later as "the big social idea" to come out of the war.

Writing to one former colleague in September 1942, Bolotin described the first months of the war: "This is all like a three-ring circus, with Washington, Richmond, and Oakland all smoothly and wonderfully performing at the same time." She called Garfield the star performer, better than any Hollywood star. She knew something historic was unfolding, writing, "'Tis like heady wine to be even a small dot in this organization." Bolotin's admiration only grew as she served as Garfield's executive assistant through the war years, writing in 1944 that "his amazing vitality, abilities, and many accomplishments are still, after three years, astounding to me. To try and keep up with him is almost too much …"

Garfield, the man who once hated the idea of becoming a doctor, now loved being a surgeon and an administrator. He never completely gave up surgery, even as wartime pushed him into his new role overseeing the explosive growth of his medical program. His administrative leadership became his new calling, poignantly remembered by Bolotin in describing how he gave up most, though not all, surgery. When a particularly difficult surgical case arrived at the hospital, she said, "the next thing I knew, Sid was upstairs doing the surgery and pulled the man through."

When Garfield returned from the surgery, Bolotin asked, "Sid, why aren't you practicing surgery, with your fantastic capabilities?"

"There are a lot of fine surgeons," he responded, "but very few people can do what I'm doing now."

Few people, indeed, could have managed so efficiently and so quickly the construction or rebuilding of major urban hospitals, while also pulling together the medical teams to staff them and shaping the financial mechanism to provide the illness prevention and care that was needed. Of course he had the help of Ordway and others from the Kaiser organization. Most important was the backing of Henry J. Kaiser. History has shown that without Kaiser's business success and clout, Garfield likely would never have succeeded in creating a huge, financially self-sufficient medical care program. Likewise, Henry Kaiser's desire to support expansion of medical care to working people would never have succeeded without Dr. Garfield's ideas.

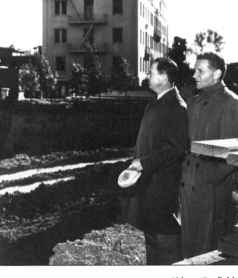

Sidney Garfield with Ned Dodds, a Kaiser employee, viewing the beginning of rehabilitation work on the old Fabiola Hospital, which would become the Permanente Foundation Hospital, in Oakland, California.

During those war years, Garfield and Kaiser forged a complex personal friendship and business partnership. A revealing story of their mutual dependence involved the financing of the Permanente Foundation Hospital in Oakland, which opened in August 1942. Garfield had purchased the abandoned four-story maternity wing of a former hospital named Fabiola; to rebuild it required a $250,000 loan.

Garfield and Kaiser went to San Francisco to meet with Kaiser's banker, A.P. Giannini, founder and president of Bank of America. Garfield explained in some detail his

41

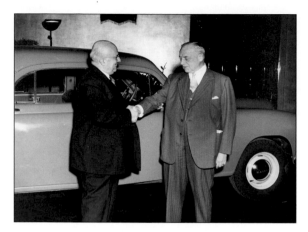

Bank of America founder A.P. Giannini and Henry J. Kaiser. Giannini, Kaiser's long-time banker, provided the crucial financing for the rebuilding of what became the Permanente Foundation Hospital in Oakland, California. Photo credit: Bank of America.

innovative ideas and unique experience, covering the history of his own program for the aqueduct workers in the Mojave Desert and what he had created for Kaiser at Grand Coulee Dam. Giannini, despite his liberal lending policy for innovative ideas, merely laughed because hospitals of the era had bad track records for paying back loans. "We won't loan a penny to hospitals," Giannini said. "They never, never can pay off and, if you try to foreclose on them, what do you do with a hospital?"

However, Kaiser had banked with Giannini since 1921, when Kaiser arrived in California. By World War II, Kaiser held the largest single line of credit in Bank of America history to that point. And Giannini liked Kaiser. He always paid his loans off on schedule — and sometimes even ahead of time. Giannini turned to Kaiser. "Henry," he said, "if you want to guarantee the loan, I'll let you have two hundred and fifty thousand." "I'll guarantee it," Kaiser replied. "We've got a record at Coulee and the doctor has had hospitals on the desert where he always paid off his debts. I think we can chance it."

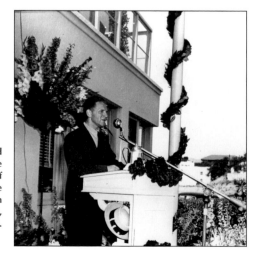

Sidney Garfield speaking at the dedication of the Permanente Foundation Hospital in Oakland, California, August 21, 1942.

With that first loan, and within a few months, Garfield opened the thoroughly modern 54-bed Permanente Foundation Hospital, which the Foundation owned and Garfield and Associates leased. More remarkable than the rapid makeover, once the hospital was in operation, Garfield repaid the loan in record time. He thereby established the financial viability of prepaid health insurance in the eyes of Giannini. For the next two decades, Sidney Garfield was the innovative idea man behind many of the new designs for Kaiser hospitals, all with financing from Bank of America in an era when banks mostly refused to loan money to hospitals.

With Oakland open, Garfield immediately swung into action to build a Permanente Foundation Hospital to serve shipyard workers in Portland and Vancouver. There, however, he got his first taste of the opposition he would face after the war from many in traditional medicine. While community physicians in Richmond and Oakland were mostly willing to tolerate Garfield's unorthodox wartime program,

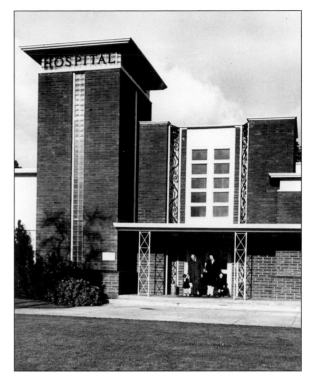

Main entrance of the Permanente Foundation Hospital in Vancouver, Washington, the first hospital built from scratch. Designed by Sidney Garfield during World War II, the innovative structure brought him national recognition.

it was partly out of fear of being overwhelmed by the sheer numbers of shipyard patients. In Portland, Garfield and Edgar Kaiser got a very different reaction. There, a leader of the community physicians bluntly told them to go across the Columbia River to the small town of Vancouver, Washington: "Do what you want over there. Nobody cares what you do." The problem was that prepayment and group medical practices threatened the financial status quo of the fee-for-service medical community. Physicians did not trust their livelihoods to a new idea and they resented any encroachment on their own practices. When Garfield, who strongly opposed the growing movement for government-supported health care, eloquently described his plan to physicians in Portland, the *Portland Oregonian* headlined its story "Socialization Plan Denied."

So it was in this context in Vancouver that Garfield — the kid who had dreamed of being an architect or engineer — had the chance to build a full-scale hospital from scratch. Ideas flowed from his experiences with his small, 12-bed hospital at Desert Center, the renovation at Mason City, the Field Hospital in Richmond, and the rebuilt Permanente Foundation Hospital in Oakland. But Garfield's most important idea was one he brought from his days as the surgical "super resident" at Los Angeles County General Hospital. Despite the new county hospital's reputation as one of the most modern in the world, Garfield grew frustrated with the 15th floor operating rooms. "The surgical suite," he concluded, "was a mess." There was a single corridor, with the operating rooms on each side of it. It was crowded with stretchers, supplies, and people. It was a hazard to walk, and it was hard to keep supplies sterile. The supervisor was at one end of the long hallway, and it took valuable time to get his or her help when needed.

Concluding that "there ought to be a better way of building surgeries than this," Garfield went out and got himself a drawing board — something he kept at hand thereafter — and began sketching ideas for a new design. His idea for a surgical suite was a circle of operating rooms, with the supervisor in the center. The space between the supervisor and the operating rooms would be a sterile supply area. To keep this interior corridor clean, Garfield drew a second, exterior corridor for removing used and contaminated materials. Orderlies now could bring the stretchers in from the outside without going through the sterile area. "I passed that design around to all our surgeons at the Los Angeles County General Hospital and they all thought that [it] was a good idea," Garfield said.

Of course, it was only an academic exercise when he was at Los Angeles County General Hospital. Now, however, Garfield had a chance to build a surgical suite of his own, although he would have to work fast. Given the wartime pressures, the Permanente Foundation Hospital in Vancouver would have patients coming through its doors in a mere three months. The design innovation attracted wide attention, drawing a steady stream of hospital planners and administrators who wanted to see it in action. They were impressed with how it saved steps, improved aseptic techniques, reduced congestion, and resulted in better controls and supervision. This would be the first of dozens of design innovations

Garfield would introduce over the next few decades, leading *Modern Hospital* magazine to once remark, "Dr. Garfield's innovations have been raising the eyebrows, and sometimes the hair, of traditionalists since the 1930s."

Garfield's reputation for innovative and revolutionary approaches to medical care continued to grow and was attracting attention and admiration far and wide. His approach to industrial medical care was increasingly supported by the United States Maritime Commission, and quickly grew into the largest civilian medical care program on the Home Front. By the spring of 1945, he had 200 hospital beds in Richmond; 134 at Oakland with another 100 under construction; 300 in Vancouver; and 45 in Fontana. Dignitaries began arriving from all over to look at this wartime medical care program. "The medical schools, industries throughout the country, individual physicians, lay people, everyone seems to have their finger pointed at us and what we are doing," Bolotin wrote in 1944. Official visitors to one or more of the Kaiser Shipyard hospitals included President and Eleanor Roosevelt, Treasury Secretary Henry Morgenthau, and Vice President Henry Wallace, among others. Other visitors included the deans of various medical schools and, Bolotin wrote to a friend, "a thousand and one other celebrities. Our guest list reads like the Blue Book or Who's Who."

To accommodate such a steady flood of prominent visitors, Garfield had to assign someone to teach Sally Bolotin how to drive. She became the tour guide of the medical care program in the Richmond Shipyards. This attention, however, was mild compared with the acclaim — and controversy — to come when Paul de Kruif, the most famous medical and science author of the era, focused his interests on Garfield. He turned Garfield — sometimes with considerable hyperbole — into the hero of a series of articles and books that would make Garfield one of the most admired — and castigated — physicians of his time.

Henry J. Kaiser's shipbuilders during World War II became famous for building ships faster than anyone in history. Whether they worked in his steel mill in Fontana, California, or in any of his shipyards in Richmond, California; Portland, Oregon; or Vancouver, Washington, today they are honored by the Rosie the Riveter / World War II Home Front National Historical Park in Richmond. So, too, is Dr. Sidney Garfield. As these shipbuilders came by the tens of thousands to the West Coast, Garfield built the largest civilian medical care program on the Home Front to promote wellness and safety among the workers as well as take care of them when they were injured or became ill. From this work was born Kaiser Permanente, with a focus on prevention, prepayment, and multispecialty group medical practice.

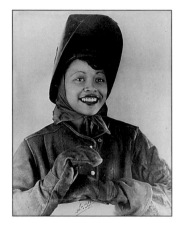

Gladys Theus was said to be "one of the fastest and most efficient welders" in the Richmond Shipyards, according to information on file with her photograph in the Franklin D. Roosevelt Presidential Library.

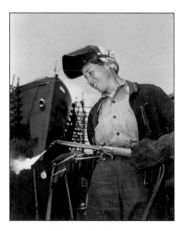

Mary Carroll of Portland, Oregon, above, and her roommate were the first two women in history hired by an American shipyard, the Kaiser operation in the Pacific Northwest. Carroll is seen in a portrait by famed Portland photographer Ray Atkeson.

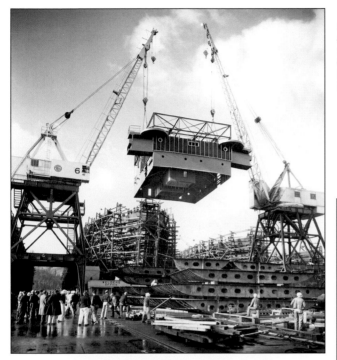

Kaiser West Coast Shipyards launched a ship a day and broke all shipbuilding records. Here (top) a prefabricated deckhouse is hoisted into place in Portland, while a ship (bottom) is launched at Richmond.

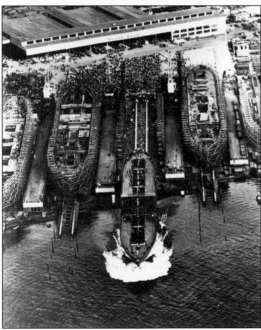

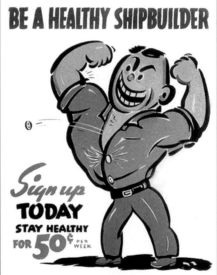

It fell to Sidney Garfield and the doctors, nurses, and other staff he hired to keep the shipyard workers healthy as they opened the Permanente Health Plan in 1942.

x

47

A nurse gives a shipyard worker first aid treatment in Richmond (below), while a child is looked after by a nurse in a pediatrics clinic in Vancouver (right) as Sidney Garfield's prepaid, prevention-focused group practice medical care program provided comprehensive services on the Home Front.

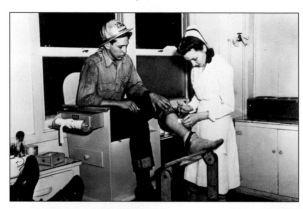

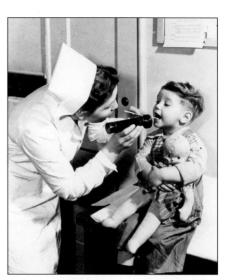

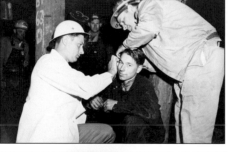

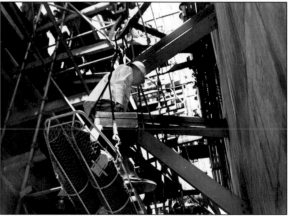

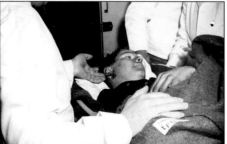

First aid crews (left middle) stood at the ready to handle injuries, (above) in this case an unidentified worker being treated at the scene of an accident and then hoisted on a stretcher to ground level for a trip to the hospital. In the final photograph, (left) a surgeon exams the injured shipbuilder at the Richmond Field Hospital, which today is a national historic site.

"Safety Pays" reads a linoleum inlay (below) at the feet of shipyard workers who wait for routine care at the Richmond First Aid Station; (right) an employee of the Vancouver Shipyard picks up a prescription at the Permanente Foundation Hospital.

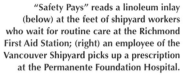

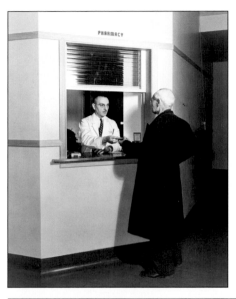

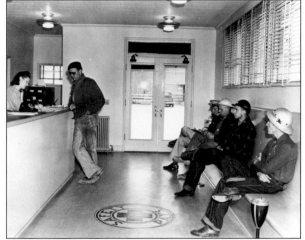

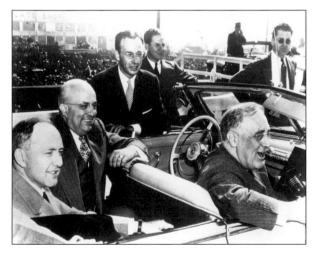

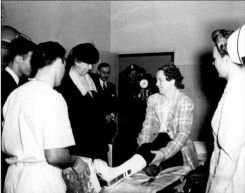

President Franklin D. Roosevelt (left) speaks to a crowd at the shipyards in Vancouver on September 23, 1942 as, from left, then Oregon Governor Charles Sprague, Henry Kaiser and his son Edgar, looked on. First Lady Eleanor Roosevelt (above) visited with an unidentified patient who has just had a cast put on her leg at the hospital in Vancouver. Sidney Garfield treasured this photograph, one of only a few of Kaiser Permanente history that he kept in his personal collection.

Chapter 7

Postwar Challenges: Rebuilding Against a Tide of Opposition

Having successfully developed the largest private, prepaid medical care program in the United States, Sidney Garfield could look back with great satisfaction and forward with equal enthusiasm. In a brief essay he wrote to mark the first anniversary of his program, published in the January 1944 issue of the *Permanente Foundation Medical Bulletin*, Garfield dared to imagine the possibilities for a fundamental transformation of American medicine in the postwar world.

Prepayment, group practice, and adequate facilities, he argued, were the essential keys to unlocking a transformation of medicine in the postwar world that could focus on keeping patients healthy, not merely treating the sick. "How much wiser to transfer the economy of medicine to payment for keeping the patient well," he said. "Such becomes the case with prepaid group medicine operating in efficient and adequate facilities. Under these conditions, the fewer the sick, the more remuneration; the less serious the illness, the better off the patient and the doctors."

Garfield aimed the appeal directly at the new generation of physicians emerging from medical schools and the young physicians who would eventually be returning from military service. These were doctors accustomed to working in close collaboration with colleagues and without personal economic interests. "Well-trained young men under the private practice system spend the best years of their lives waiting to be discovered," he warned. Possibly remembering his own self-exile to the desert and to primary care medicine as a young surgeon, he added: "During this period they are disillusioned and often forced to step beyond their fields and ability because of financial reasons. Such a man entering a group could immediately be used to his full capacity, because under such a system the group sponsors the young man." Organized on a statewide basis, preferably by the doctors of the state medical association, Garfield argued that such a system could accommodate private practice, group practice, and even a mixture of the two, benefiting patients with genuine "health" care, in addition to sick care. It could also put the postwar medical profession on a more stable, rewarding, and ethical foundation — and all without resorting to any sort of government-provided health care.

Later in 1944, while participating on an expert panel on prepaid plans at the annual session of the AMA in Chicago, Garfield carried the same message to an audience of highly skeptical AMA colleagues (Appendix 1). What was needed to defeat the growing political movement for government-managed national health insurance, he said, was for the AMA's county and state-level medical associations to form their own group practices and embrace prepaid, comprehensive insurance, as demonstrated

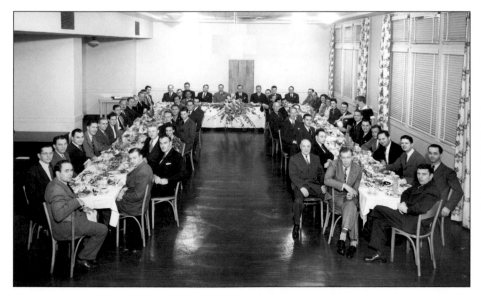

The Sidney Garfield and Associates medical group dinner in 1944, hosted by Garfield. Within a year, the end of World War II would threaten the continued existence of the medical group and the entire medical care program.

by the success of the Permanente program at the Kaiser Shipyards. "I can honestly say that the only thing wrong with what we are doing," he said, "is that neither Mr. Kaiser nor I should be doing it. The doctors, through their medical organizations, should be doing the job. If they would they could raise American medicine far beyond its present level ... and, what is more important, bring it to the people."

If anyone needed proof of the manifold advantages of such a system, they had only to look to what had been accomplished in a few short years, under wartime conditions, in the West Coast Shipyards. The story of that medical miracle had been documented and widely publicized in a series of articles in *Reader's Digest*, published in book form in 1943 as *Kaiser Wakes the Doctors*, by Paul de Kruif. De Kruif, a microbiologist best known for his 1926 book, *The Microbe Hunters*, had been urged by Henry Kaiser to come to California and have a firsthand look at the medical program that Garfield was building to serve the Richmond Shipyards. He came, he saw, and he stayed, virtually embedding himself among Garfield's eager doctors and grateful, working-class patients. De Kruif celebrated the Permanente program as a "community Mayo Clinic for the common man" that sought "to bring maximum medical care within the reach of all the people, to keep medicine in the hands of the doctors and the people, and to keep medicine out of the hands of government bureaucrats." The book was a top seller, with multiple editions, including a British edition that offered Garfield's approach as a private enterprise alternative to the government-run health care system then being debated in England.

Reader's Digest wasn't the only periodical taking approving notice. Although the medical mainstream, in the form of the AMA and its vituperative, longtime journal editor, Morris Fishbein, continued to rail against all forms of prepayment and group practice as "socialized medicine," the prestigious *New England Journal of Medicine* (*NEJM*) editorialized on Garfield's first anniversary essay shortly after it appeared. It noted that it "makes impressive reading and merits more than a glance by physicians who are interested in the socioeconomic aspects of medical practice. Those who are actively concerned with the problems of prepaid health and medical care insurance may find it useful to adopt some of these methods and principles in order to bring the most effective and efficient medical service to large numbers of people at low cost — and at the same time to maintain the high standards and dignity of the medical profession." Finally, at least some quarters of the medical profession were willing to glimpse and acknowledge the promising postwar possibilities that Garfield was pioneering and preaching.

The sense of satisfaction didn't last long. A mere year later, all those possibilities must have seemed to Garfield and his closest colleagues more distant than ever. The promise of peace threatened, ironically, to wipe away the promise of a new medical future. With the end of World War II and government support for Home Front jobs, the Richmond Shipyard workforce plummeted in a matter of months from 90,000 to about 10,000. Similar reductions occurred at the Portland/Vancouver operations. In Oakland, Garfield's medical group, Sidney Garfield and Associates, dropped from about 100 physicians to a mere dozen, while the group in Vancouver moved to shut down the entire medical program.

"I never thought they would shut the shipyards down overnight," Garfield later recalled. "I didn't think that was possible … We lost our membership. Most of them returned from whence they came, from all parts of the country."

As Dr. John Smillie noted in his history of the early years of Permanente (*Can Physicians Manage the Quality and Costs of Health Care?* New York: McGraw-Hill, 1991*),* "Prepaid group medical practice seemed once again to be — in the words of the wartime bureaucracy (which assigned physicians to Garfield) — stamped 'for the duration only.'"

But Garfield, it turned out, was wrong about one thing. The departing shipyard workforce did not return "from whence they came" when the shipyards closed down. A large percentage of them stayed in the Bay Area and the Portland area, and many, along with returning veterans, gravitated into the growing ranks of West Coast industrial unions as the California population — and economy — exploded over the coming decade. They would come to represent one of the essential ingredients that Garfield's programs in the Mojave Desert and at Grand Coulee lacked — a large, geographically concentrated source of potential members not affiliated with a temporary industrial enterprise, such as an aqueduct, dam, or wartime shipyard. What's more, they were already familiar with and appreciative of the prepaid group practice model of medical care — an alien form of medicine in much of the country.

In most other respects, Garfield was foresighted about the future. Well before the war ended so suddenly, he and his close colleague, Cecil Cutting, M.D., had enlisted the help of a Kaiser executive, Eugene Trefethen, in plotting a strategy to transform the wartime industrial medical program into a postwar public program, open to all comers. Acknowledging the need to continue to provide care for some 10,000 postwar Kaiser Shipyard workers, Trefethen agreed to create a new nonprofit trust, known as the Permanente Health Plan, as of September 1945 to enroll those and other members in a public program. This new trust was in addition to the Permanente Foundation, created in 1942 for operation of the wartime hospitals and medical care. Garfield would serve as sole proprietor of the much-diminished medical group, which would lease the existing hospitals from the Permanente Foundation, a nonprofit holding company. He would also act as executive director over the entire tripartite enterprise.

Now, with a nonprofit health plan in place to blunt potential criticisms about the corporate practice of medicine (or doctors working under the tutelage of for-profit corporations run by lay businessmen), all that was needed was capital for new and modernized facilities, new members to replace the tens of thousands of departed shipyard workers, and new doctors sympathetic to the prepaid group practice model. The challenges were daunting, even for leaders with the visionary and organizational zeal of Garfield and Kaiser.

Fortunately, Garfield had had the foresight during the war to set aside a portion of the money paid to his medical group by the insurance companies, expressly for postwar conversion. That contingency fund now amounted to $1.5 million. To generate additional revenue, the Health Plan instituted small copays to supplement the insurance premiums. Garfield instituted his so-called "economy of shortages" — a policy of maximizing the cost-effectiveness of everything from hospital beds to physician productivity by keeping all resources at the minimum levels needed for quality patient care. He also promoted a strict culture of economy throughout the organization by repairing rather than replacing broken furniture, personally reviewing all expenditures, and among other economies, requiring employees to turn in three-inch pencil stubs in order to get a new pencil. These policies evolved into a lasting Permanente culture emphasizing the efficient allocation of medical resources that continues to this day.

Membership growth, beyond the 10,000 remaining Kaiser Shipyard workers, was a particular challenge because of the then-longtime professional prohibition against advertising or soliciting patients. As it turned out, the Health Plan grew rapidly without marketing, thanks initially to loyal former shipyard workers who wanted the plan to survive and enlisted their friends and coworkers to join, even going so far as to collect and submit regular dues from their cohorts.

The most significant growth, however, came not from individual members but from groups — faculty associations, civil service workers, and especially local unions. They became enthusiastic backers of the Permanente emphasis on preventive health screenings, primary care through ambulatory clinics, and comprehensive care for all social sectors. The organized employees of the City of Oakland were the first to sign up, joined soon after by federal civilian employees at the Alameda Naval Air Station. University of California at Berkeley and San Francisco State University faculty signed on, as did Berkeley city school employees, the East Bay Municipal Utility District workers, unionized milk wagon drivers, typographers, street car drivers and carpenters. In the first six months of operation of the public plan, new members poured in at the rate of 2,000 a month. In early 1946, the Alameda County Central Labor Council announced support for the Permanente Health Plan and the unionized Permanente

Foundation Hospital. "The endorsement for the plan by the Council will undoubtedly encourage other unions to study the plan and make it available to their membership," said the council in announcing the support. "It is to be noted that the Permanente Hospital is the only hospital in this area which is fully unionized and, if only for that reason alone, deserves the support of labor. In addition, this Health Plan is based on several principles which make good sense to a union man."

The growth continued at an astonishing rate throughout the late 1940s, so that by the turn of the decade the Permanente Health Plan in northern California boasted 120,000 members, including more than 900 employee groups. In southern California, membership more than tripled from 3,000 to 10,000, and the Portland/Vancouver plan went from nearly none to 23,000. In that same year, 1950, Harry Bridges, leader of the sprawling West Coast International Longshoremen and Warehousemen Union (ILWU), brought his entire membership of nearly 6,000 workers into Permanente — nearly 15,000 new members, including dependents. A year later, Retail Clerks Union Local 770 in Los Angeles signed on, bringing in 30,000 new members and giving Permanente a firm foothold in Los Angeles proper, where a new 200-bed Permanente Hospital opened in 1953.

In 1952, as Garfield looked back over the first decade of the Permanente medical care program in his 10th Anniversary Report (Appendix 2), he could boast of historic success on all fronts. The program had gone from near death at the end of the war to 250,000 members, including 160,000 in northern California. The Permanente Medical Group, formed out of the old Sidney Garfield and Associates group in 1948, had 125 physicians — the largest civilian medical group in the country. The nonprofit Permanente Hospitals included four major hospitals, with three more under construction in Los Angeles, San Francisco, and Walnut Creek, in addition to a number of outpatient clinics.

More importantly, the vision of prepaid group practice medicine was no longer just an aspiration; it was a firmly established reality in American medicine, here to stay. "The accolade of 'mission accomplished' cannot be too far off," wrote Garfield.

⊰ Chapter 8 ⊱

Attack from the Rear Guard

The challenges to building — and then rebuilding — a firm foundation for this new model of medical care were not merely matters of financing operations and winning over a loyal membership, however. Even as Garfield surveyed his accomplishments in 1952, more invidious challenges that had dogged him at every step persisted. Strident opposition from the old guard medical mainstream was now increasingly abetted by Cold War suspicions of leftist unions, like the ILWU, and their partners.

In fact, the physician opposition to prepaid comprehensive insurance and group practice medicine predated the Permanente program by at least a decade. As early as 1932, when the prestigious Committee on the Costs of Medical Care issued its 23-volume report, urging adoption of both prepayment and group practice, Morris Fishbein, the powerful "voice of the AMA" and longtime editor of the *Journal of the American Medical Association* (*JAMA*), labeled the report "socialism and communism, inciting to revolution." Two years later, he noted with approval that the AMA's Los Angeles County association had expelled Drs. Donald Ross and H. Clifford Loos, founders of the Ross-Loos Medical Group, from the society on charges of soliciting patients, among other offenses. Ross and Loos had been running a prepaid group practice program for the Los Angeles Department of

Water and Power's 12,000 industrial workers. It was not far — but, fortunately, far enough — from Garfield's Contractors General Hospital in the Mojave Desert, which escaped the society's notice thanks to its remoteness. In his monthly *JAMA* column, entitled "Mr. Pepys' Diary," which ran for nearly 25 years, Fishbein never missed an opportunity to castigate by name as "unethical" and "socialistic" anyone who dared suggest reforms of the solo practice, fee-for-service medical status quo. And he strongly backed the actions of state and county associations in their efforts to prevent prepayment and group practice advocates from practicing medicine by denying them association membership. This, in turn, made it nearly impossible for such doctors to get hospital privileges, patient referrals, or specialty society accreditation. The tactics persisted even after the U.S. Supreme Court ruled in 1943 that the AMA and its District of Columbia association were guilty of restraint of trade against physicians of the prepaid group practice, Group Health Association of Washington, DC, under the terms of the Sherman Antitrust Act. That ruling prompted more antitrust suits against the AMA, including a successful action against the King County Medical Association in Seattle for denying membership to the physicians of the Group Health Cooperative of Puget Sound, whose prepaid medical group would much later assume the name Permanente and become part of The Permanente Federation, although not part of the overall Kaiser Permanente system.

Adding fuel to the fire of AMA opposition, increasingly strong political forces at both the national and state levels were pressing for legislation to create compulsory health insurance programs, organized by the government. The AMA built up a massive war chest to oppose these efforts throughout the mid-1940s and into the 1950s. During this time, California legislators mounted five separate campaigns for statewide insurance programs.

For the most part, Garfield was spared mainstream medicine's strident opposition to insurance reform and prepaid group practice during the 1930s and early 1940s. His medical care programs in the desert and at Grand Coulee were remote, self-contained industrial care operations, just outside the radar of mainstream medicine. Even the World War II Home Front programs failed to draw much attention from the association, since they were confined to shipyard workers and their dependents. They were limited, in the official jargon, to operations "for the duration" of the war. An exception was the situation in the Portland/Vancouver area, where the Northern Permanente Foundation ran into opposition to their recruitment of community physicians from the Seattle Medical Society, which controlled the wartime assignment of physicians in the region. Garfield traveled north and made personal, friendly appeals to the society, only to be allocated the least productive and least competent physicians in the community. "They (society leaders) were friendly to me," Garfield recalled, "but they'd say, 'This guy is no damn good. You take him. We don't care what you do with him.'"

The attitude of benign neglect, however, lasted only "for the duration." Once the war was over and the Permanente programs opened their doors to public membership in mid-1945, Garfield and, increasingly, Henry Kaiser became big game in the scopes of the AMA and its local associations. They viewed an expanding, urbanized, public Permanente as both a dire competitive threat and an ideological assault on the tradition of fee-for-service, open choice, solo-practice medicine under the control of physicians, not laymen. To the medical mainstream, Permanente looked like the antithesis of that tradition, especially as the medical group appeared to be under the pay and control of the Permanente Health Plan, technically controlled by a board of trustees made up of executives of Kaiser Industries.

The assault on Permanente began in earnest in mid-1946, just a year after going public. The Ethics Committee of the Alameda County Medical Association lodged a complaint before the state Board of Medical Examiners charging Garfield with employing unlicensed physicians, specifically a resident and a physician whose license was on probation.

The first case involved Dr. Clifford Keene, a highly qualified Army surgeon and former chief resident at the University of Michigan Hospital. Garfield had hired him to run a medical facility at a Kaiser automobile plant in Willow Run, Michigan, where he was licensed. But Garfield wanted to check out Keene's capabilities for a short time at Oakland before dispatching him to Michigan. Knowing Keene had no California license, Garfield put him on staff as a temporary resident for three months, because interns and residents not only did not require a license, but could not be licensed until completing their training. (Keene, who had since left for Michigan, would return to Oakland during the investigation, pass the California medical exam, and go on to play a major, if not medical, role in the future of Kaiser Permanente.)

The other case involved an emergency medicine physician, Thomas Flint, Jr., who, before joining Permanente, had been put on probation by the Medical Examiners Board for self-administering a narcotic drug as a pain killer. This fact was known to Cecil Cutting, chief of staff at the Permanente Hospital, who made a point of obtaining permission to hire him from the chairman of the Medical Examiners Board. But that permission had never been conveyed to the full board for approval.

In any community hospital, such cases would have drawn little if any attention, and certainly no official censure. But this was no community hospital; this was Permanente, the prime offender against some of the most hidebound traditions of American medicine. Thus, although the complaint involving Flint was dropped (the Board chairman, after all, had approved his hiring), the charge involving Keene was sustained. The Board suspended Garfield's license to practice medicine for one year and placed him on five-year probation — a devastating setback for the leader of a medical group in the process of postwar rebuilding. Garfield promptly went to court to fight the suspension and won a judgment against the Medical Examiners Board, but the damage was done. Fishbein's *JAMA* reported that Garfield's license had been suspended, neglecting to note the suspension had been stayed. And the *Oakland Tribune* added to its report that the county medical association was accusing the Permanente Foundation and Hospital of "a production line type of medical care."

Meanwhile, the Bay Area county medical societies stepped up the campaign against other Permanente physicians by denying them society membership. This tactic was aimed at discouraging community physicians from joining Permanente, since doing so would limit their ability to ever return to the fee-for-service medical community if Permanente should fail. When even this failed to slow the rapid growth of Permanente membership in the East Bay and San Francisco — in stark contrast to the struggling solo practices in a postwar Bay Area market suffering a growing oversupply of physicians — the Council of the Alameda County Medical Society readied a second assault on Garfield.

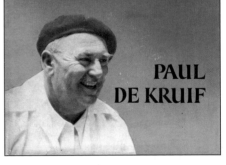

Alerted that further, unknown medical ethics charges were pending, Garfield sought help in building whatever defense might be required by calling on his wartime public relations champion, journalist Paul de Kruif and his wife, Rhea.

"Sid phoned us long distance, with no preliminary explanations, asking us how quick we could get out to the Coast," de Kruif recalled in his subsequent book, *Life Among the Doctors,* (New York: Harcourt Brace, 1949). Three days later, Garfield picked up the de Kruifs at the Mills Field airport south of San Francisco. Over the following months, de Kruif would produce a second series of glowing articles on Garfield and his program, along with condemnations of his opponents, for the millions of readers of *Reader's Digest*. "It seemed Sid's crime," wrote de Kruif, "was that of building a pilot plan for good medical care within the means of the ordinary citizen, paying its own way without charity or government socialization. For this, Sid was to be tried by the doctors as unethical …"

Paul de Kruif, pictured on the cover of his book *Life Among the Doctors,* offered the most detailed account of the attack against Sidney Garfield by the mainstream medical establishment of the 1940s.

The anticipated second attack on Garfield also roused his friend and partner, Henry Kaiser, to action. After all, apart from wanting to protect Garfield's reputation, his own reputation was now at stake, since he was increasingly identified with the medical care program. Any attack on Permanente on ethical grounds was an attack on Kaiser's own integrity. In a lengthy broadside sent to a Bay Area newspaper, he wrote, "Those who know Dr. Garfield will be forever grateful, as I am, to Dr. Garfield and his staff for the great service they have rendered the community at great personal sacrifice. It is quite possible that there are those in our western cities who don't want to see Dr. Garfield suffer, but who are falsely represented by the small but vocally strong minority interests who are fighting to destroy our plan of prepaid medicine."

In discussions with de Kruif, Garfield pondered what the exact charges against him might be, assuming that the aim was to "chuck him out of the medical association for not meeting the health needs of the patients." De Kruif responded: "Wait a minute. Hold it! What's the ultimate index of health needs, Sid? Death rates. What about Permanente's death rates in large series of cases of specific ailments, in large series of operations — do you have them?" Assured that such data was available, de Kruif suggested compiling mortality rates comparing Permanente to other hospitals in the Bay Area and the state.

For the next week, everyone scurried about to compile mortality rates for the Permanente Foundation Hospital, San Francisco County Hospital, the University of California Service and Los Angeles County General Hospital, among others. Hopefully, de Kruif reasoned, the local doctors would call off the pending attack if they realized that Permanente's rates compared favorably with those of their own hospitals. As it turned out, the comparisons provided ample ammunition, should they choose to use it. Deaths from pneumococcal lobar pneumonia, a common condition during the war years, were radically lower at the Permanente Foundation Hospital than those at the University of California Service across the bay in the San Francisco County Hospital, for instance. Mortality for perforated peptic ulcer at Permanente was the lowest of 32 comparable series nationwide, including those at San Francisco County Hospital and Los Angeles County General Hospital.

Kaiser, nonetheless, seemed wary of the prospect of an open battle. During a weekend retreat at his estate at Lake Tahoe, Kaiser and the de Kruifs pondered their strategy. "All that weekend, banging us about in his very fast speedboats on Lake Tahoe, sitting before the big fire in our guesthouse at Homewood (a nearby resort village) … the big man thought out loud, fumbling at the thorny problem … How could he fix it so that Permanente and solo (practice) medicine could live side-by-side — maybe even cooperating," wrote de Kruif. "I have never seen the genial giant so serious or sad as he was that week."

The following Tuesday, June 8, 1948, a letter arrived via special delivery. It contained the charges of the Alameda County Medical Association. They included "advertising and solicitation of patients" for the health plan, putting "mass production techniques" before patient needs, preventing free choice of physicians, rendering inadequate service at an understaffed hospital, and diverting illegal and unethical profits into the nonprofit Permanente Foundation. It even repeated the prior charge of employing "unlicensed personnel."

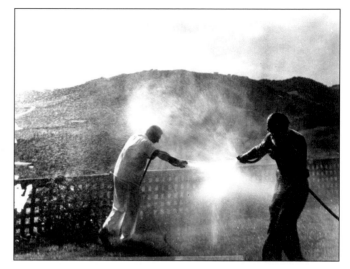

Though times were trying, Sidney Garfield and his old friend and associate Cecil Cutting still found time to relax and enjoy themselves at Cutting's home in Orinda, California.

While Garfield pondered how to respond, Kaiser, "astounded and horrified," according to de Kruif, went on the offensive. In a meeting with local community physicians at the St. Francis Hotel in San Francisco, he expressed himself as "profoundly shocked" that "a group of Alameda County doctors [would declare] war on the Permanente Health program," which he described as the only alternative to "government medicine." According to historian Ricky Hendricks, author of a book-length history of Kaiser Permanente, (A *Model for National Health Care: A History of Kaiser Permanente,* New Brunswick, NJ: Rutgers University Press, 1993), Kaiser reminded them of the 1943 Supreme Court's restraint of trade ruling against the AMA and told them, "If, as we believe, a conspiracy to restrain the practice of medicine exists, the state of California is by law obligated to proceed with dissolution of the medical associations." Backing off from open warfare, he proposed the doctors should agree to a "spirit of peace" and help implement prepaid group practice medicine as an alternative to the threat of a national health plan — a strategy Kaiser and his team of advisors had agreed to in a meeting the previous evening.

Once the outrage passed, Garfield, Kaiser, the de Kruifs and their legal counsel settled on a less aggressive, less public strategy. Noting that no member of the medical society leadership had ever, as far as anyone knew, stepped foot in the Permanente Hospital or otherwise examined its operations to determine the accuracy of the charges, they decided to invite them in for an open look. Whatever they wanted to see, including the financial records, would be open to them without restriction. The society accepted the invitation and promised not to put Garfield on trial until the investigation was complete.

Over the following year, several committees of local physicians visited the Permanente Hospital, examined records, and interviewed physicians. They also let it be known, according to Cecil Cutting, that the whole mess could be swept away if the local community doctors were allowed to treat Permanente members and be reimbursed on a fee-for-service basis by the Permanente Health Plan — "a less than subtle form of shakedown," as Permanente historian John Smillie, M.D., called it.

The investigations turned up no evidence of poor quality care, profiteering, or understaffing. In fact, the final report was fairly glowing in its description of the care rendered by Permanente, and a number of participating community physicians were won over to outright support for Permanente. But there was one minor exception. Apparently, $61,000 had been budgeted by the Health Plan for "promotion and selling" during a short period in 1945, thus giving some substance to the charge of soliciting for patients. But since that practice had never been repeated, that charge, along with all the others, was found to be without merit. In November 1949, the Alameda County Medical Association withdrew all charges against Garfield.

Nonetheless, the intense focus of the campaign against Garfield had important organizational and perhaps personal repercussions. For one thing, Garfield's brief, two-year marriage to Virginia Jackson, a talented Permanente nurse, dissolved in 1948 as Ginny fell prey to alcoholism. While there is no evidence that the marriage problems had anything to do with attacks on Garfield, the breakdown of the marriage must certainly have added to the intense pressures he was feeling. Also, to defuse the attacks on himself as the embodiment of Permanente, Garfield agreed in February 1948 to a reorganization of the overall program that included dissolving the Sidney Garfield and Associates medical group, of which he was sole proprietor. The medical group was reconstituted as a partnership called The Permanente Medical Group, with seven original full partners, including Garfield, who received no compensation for Sidney Garfield and Associates. But even that was not enough to remove him from the spotlight, since he was now vulnerable to attack for being a partner in a for-profit medical group while acting as executive officer of the nonprofit Permanente Health Plan and the nonprofit Hospitals organization.

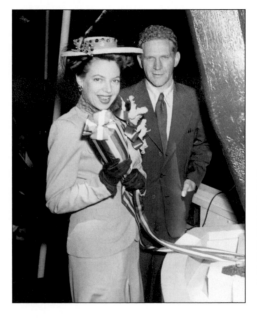

Sidney Garfield's first wife, Virginia, prepares to christen the William Allen White at the Kaiser Shipyards in Richmond, California, 1944.

Thus, on July 1, 1949, five months before the Medical Association dropped the charges against him, a new The Permanente Medical Group partnership was drawn up, without Garfield as a partner. "As soon as I got out of that position, being the boss of the medical group … I had no official status," he recalled. "Then there was no longer any real reason for their attacking me. When you attack 50 different doctors, you are getting into a different sort of deal than when you are attacking only one person."

While the sacrifice of losing his medical group must have stung, Garfield, typically, was reticent to show any self-pity. "With that change," he wrote, "I divested myself of ownership and became an employee of the medical group, the health plan, and the hospitals, as the (employed) medical director of all three. I did this with complete faith — I guess you would call it blind faith — that these changes would not alter the situation that existed when I owned it. We doctors had conceived the plan, developed it, sacrificed for it, made it work, and believed that it was going to remain our operation."

Was that faith justified? Events over the next half dozen years would put that question to the test.

In the meantime, in the struggle to gain acceptance by mainstream medicine, there would be more battles to come — mostly focusing on Henry Kaiser, who took an increasingly high profile role as defender of the medical care program (a fact which the The Permanente Medical Group physicians deeply resented, as he was a layman). But as the battles wore on, it would become ever clearer that the medical societies were fighting a losing war. By June 1948, even the AMA House of Delegates finally approved a resolution, repeatedly submitted in recent years, to silence "Dr. AMA," Morris Fishbein, the voice of American medicine who had never actually practiced medicine. He was removed as editor of *JAMA* and forbidden to speak, write, or be interviewed on "controversial subjects" as long as he was associated with the AMA. His constant tirades against prepayment and group practice had become so tiresome and embarrassing that even the conservative majority of the House of Delegates, who remained fierce opponents of government reform schemes and champions of fee-for-service, solo practice medicine, viewed him as an obstacle.

As history ticked past the mid-century mark, the tide of American medicine was shifting. The old fee-for-service world seemed to many to be ebbing, with prepayment and group practice rising. And Kaiser Permanente, as the program was soon to be known, was very much in the vanguard of this new medical world.

❦ Chapter 9 ❦

Prosperity in the Postwar Boom

Of the significant things Sidney Garfield did in starting his medical care program, perhaps the most important was to convince Henry Kaiser to set up the not-for-profit Permanente Foundation as a charitable trust in 1942, at the outset of the Richmond/ Oakland program. It was revolutionary as a financing mechanism because, unlike endowed foundations, it was funded by the revenue stream of health plan members' dues. It also helped establish research as a cornerstone of Garfield's overall health care delivery system. The foundation-funded research program would evolve in the 1950s into a critical element of medical care and a basic principle of what would come to be known as Permanente Medicine.

Although Henry Kaiser, his wife, Bess, and various Kaiser Company executives made up the board of trustees of the Permanente Foundation, the concept came from doctors. Garfield's old friend and colleague from Los Angeles County General Hospital, Ray Kay, M.D., first presented the idea to Garfield. Before the U.S. entered World War II, Kay had been dispatched by the dean of the USC School of Medicine to New York to investigate foundation structures and procedures to analyze how they might be applied to medicine. In January 1942, after Garfield had agreed to stay on the Home Front to care for Kaiser's shipyard workers, he and Kay had a farewell dinner in San Francisco before Kay shipped out for Burma.

Kay shared with Garfield what he had learned about foundations. He suggested that such an entity could work as both a hospital holding company and a place to build a reserve fund for starting a prepaid group medical practice in Los Angeles after the war — an idea they had often discussed. Garfield took the idea to Clay Bedford, the Richmond Shipyard executive. He liked it and urged Garfield to take it up with Henry Kaiser, who, because his wife preferred trains to airplanes, was on board the City of San Francisco, returning to Oakland from a trip to Washington, D.C. The train would stop at Sacramento's downtown I Street station, so Bedford called for a car and driver to take Garfield the 90 miles to Sacramento. Garfield boarded the train and explained the foundation idea to Kaiser during the two-hour train ride back to Oakland. Kaiser loved the concept. However, Paul Marrin, his lawyer who was traveling with him, insisted that foundations had to be created through philanthropy, not a revenue stream, as Garfield proposed.

"It can't be done," the attorney insisted.

"Why can't it be done?" Kaiser asked.

"Well, you're not contributing any funds to the foundation. You're trying to build up a foundation out of the earnings of an operation, and that's never been done. You can't build up a foundation by its bootstraps."

Telling Henry Kaiser, the "can-do" industrialist, something was impossible was rarely a good idea. There was some argument from both Kaiser and Garfield, but Kaiser abruptly ended any debate. "Paul," he said, "I'm sick and tired of having lawyers tell me things we can't do. Now you tell me how we can do it. That's your job."

Marrin took the matter to the tax specialists at Thelen, Marrin, Johnson and Bridges, his firm in San Francisco. Six months later, papers were filed in Alameda County establishing the Permanente Foundation, a charitable trust. It was so named, at Bess Kaiser's suggestion, after a beautiful wild creek on the San Francisco Peninsula, on the bank of which the Kaisers had a private retreat. The Spanish name — Permanente Creek — came from the fact it had a year-round flow of water, unlike many in California that dry up in the arid summers.

Kaiser and Garfield took the opportunity to broaden the goals of the new foundation.

It took over ownership and the liabilities of the hospital, for which Sidney Garfield and Associates was compensated, and, in turn, leased it back to Garfield. From prepaid dues it collected, the Permanente Foundation paid for the medical care of health plan members and accumulated funds for such charitable purposes as medical research and the extension of medical services to larger populations. In short, it was to benefit both the members who joined the Permanente Foundation Health Plan and their communities. The idea that research would be a tool to bring advances in medicine to the plan's dues-paying members thus was imbedded in the medical care program from the outset. Indeed, the emphasis on research was one of the key themes in speeches at the dedication of the Oakland hospital in the fall of 1942. Henry Kaiser himself drove home the theme in his speech to the National Association of Manufacturers that December, reciting the health plan's goal to "bring not only the skill and facilities but all the advantages of research within the reach of the common man."

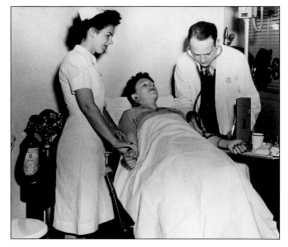

Dr. Morris Collen and a nurse checking a patient's blood pressure at the Oakland hospital, 1942.

That vision became reality starting with the work of Morris F. (Morrie) Collen, a young resident at Los Angeles County General Hospital whose dream of a career in academic medicine was on hold because of World War II. Turned down for military service because of his bronchial asthma, Collen was pondering what he was going to do when a colleague, Dr. Irv Weisenfeld, asked him if he knew that Garfield was setting up a medical care program for the Richmond Shipyards.

Feeling he had nothing to lose, Collen joined Weisenfeld for a drive to San Francisco, where they lunched with Garfield in the Garden Room of the St. Francis Hotel. A few months later, in July 1942, Collen went to work for Garfield. Once at Oakland, Collen launched the *Permanente Foundation Medical Bulletin,* which he edited for 10 years. Like other medical journals, it was distributed to medical schools and others in the medical community. Physicians reported on care of the shipyard workers, their injuries and illnesses, creating a remarkable documentary record of medicine on the Home Front of World War II. Collen, for example, treated lobar pneumonia patients from the shipyards in what turned into the largest group of patients to receive antibiotic therapy up to that point in history.

In late 1943, Collen described management of 517 pneumonia cases in the *Permanente Foundation Medical Bulletin.* Later, he wrote up the epidemiology and management of 864 additional pneumonia cases. This work caught the attention of the *New England Journal of Medicine,* which observed that the "…low fatality rates…reflects the fine type of medical care that these patients received." By 1948, the reputation of the Permanente program had grown to such prominence that interns from the University of California's medical school in San Francisco were rotating through the Permanente Foundation Hospital.

While Collen and the *Permanente Federation Medical Bulletin's* reports on clinical innovations and accomplishments heightened the program's reputation for quality medicine in the postwar years, the key to its expansion and sustained success came from a more unlikely source — organized labor.

When Harry Bridges brought his 6,000 International Longshoremen and Warehousemen Union members and their nearly 9,000 dependents to the health plan in 1950, he presented Garfield with what was as much a challenge as an opportunity: Bridges had some tough conditions in terms of where the program would need to evolve both medically and geographically. First, the offer of 15,000 new members came on condition that the plan would take on the entire ILWU membership, not only in the San Francisco Bay Area, but also in Los Angeles, San Diego, Seattle, and Portland, Oregon — regions where Permanente was little more than a hope and a dream in the minds of its physician founders.

Garfield started figuring out how to handle the influx. The San Francisco and Portland-Vancouver communities could accommodate the ILWU members with the existing health plan and facilities in both locales. Group Health Cooperative of Puget Sound, founded in 1947 as a consumer-governed, nonprofit health care system, agreed to care for them in Seattle. Similarly, an existing small health plan agreed to care for them at the port of San Diego. Los Angeles was another matter.

Garfield's biggest challenge was how to serve ILWU members in San Pedro, the port for

Los Angeles that was 25 miles southwest of downtown. The eight-doctor medical group and the 60-bed Permanente Foundation Hospital in Fontana were located 70 miles inland from San Pedro. But the opportunity to plant a sapling of the Permanente program in Garfield's adopted hometown of Los Angeles was too great to pass up. As John Smillie, M.D., wrote in his history of Kaiser Permanente, "Sidney Garfield had remained a citizen of that city. He had gone to school there. He had served his surgical residency there at the County Hospital, where he first developed a taste for group practice. He had returned to Los Angeles after the Mojave and Grand Coulee programs had ended. He had business interests there. His family still lived there, and it was in Los Angeles that he had formed some of his most enduring friendships." What's more, Garfield had not forgotten that he had promised Ray Kay, who was now at Fontana, that they would bring prepaid group medical practice to Los Angeles after the war. And so, using rented space in a medical office building in San Pedro, Garfield put a newly hired physician from Fontana, Ira Wallin, in charge of the San Pedro program. A second presence was established in southern California.

The ILWU contract with Garfield's health plan proved essential to its postwar success in more ways than one. Harry Bridges's commitment to preventive medicine meshed perfectly with Garfield's own prevention philosophy. This commitment helped set a research agenda that would influence the development and use of medical data and medical records — from early computer experiments in the 1960s to electronic medical records in the early 21st century. However, in the beginning, Bridges's insistence that his thousands of union members receive regular medical examinations presented a logistical nightmare of supply and demand.

Garfield, fortunately, was aware of the work of Dr. Lester Breslow, an emerging leader in public health who would go on to become Director of Public Health for the State of California and Dean of the School of Public Health at UCLA, and take on other key positions. In the late 1940s, Breslow recognized how inefficient medical practice was at detecting chronic diseases. So he developed and tested what he called a "multiphasic screening" approach.

Breslow noted that "early detection, early diagnosis and adequate treatment" were fundamental to preventive medicine. Yet periodic and comprehensive health examinations of large segments of the population were impractical because of the shortage of trained medical professionals in postwar America. Breslow proposed creating his multiphasic screening approach using such tools as chest X-rays, serologic testing and newly developed screening techniques for early detection of diabetes, heart disease, and some cancers. The job, he theorized, could be done using technical assistants and laboratory technicians. "Only an insignificant amount of physicians' time is required for interpretation of each person's test, especially where physicians qualified in particular screening techniques interpret the test results," he told members of the American Public Health Association in 1949. He described a trial project he developed in multiphasic screening in San Jose, California, with 954 individuals that turned up 13 cases of previously undiagnosed significant disease. He also stressed that "the multiphasic screening procedure is not a substitute for a visit to a physician."

Faced with the ILWU demand for mass screening of its members and the same shortage of personnel as everyone else, Garfield asked Morrie Collen to go talk to Breslow. "Find out from him what he's doing and how we can apply it." Collen paid Breslow a visit and was impressed with the multiphasic approach, concluding it "was very efficient in patient time and very cost effective from the viewpoint of providers." He returned to Oakland and recommended starting such a program as a major part of the solution to the ILWU membership influx and Bridges's desire for periodic health examinations. That done, another challenge remained: how to get the workers, most of whom distrusted doctors, to show up for a medical exam. Bridges's own solution was typical of his character: Bring the medical exam to the workers, right there on the waterfront. Collen accepted the challenge. "I went right down to the dock and set up simple multiphasic screening," Collen later recalled. "We collected urine specimens. We drew a blood specimen, whatever we could do there, and then took the specimens back to the Oakland Hospital laboratory, did the reports, and called in people with abnormalities."

The new program, located in the ILWU hall on Pier 18 south of San Francisco's famous

Ferry Building, was a huge hit. State and city health departments joined in, helping set up a large program run by Richard Weinerman, a young Yale-trained physician hired by Garfield as medical director of the Permanente Health Plan. Union officers were partners in helping to round up community support. The San Francisco Tuberculosis Association provided the X-ray machine and technicians. San Francisco State College provided an audiometer operator for hearing tests. The School of Public Health at the University of California at Berkeley helped out with the laboratory work. Most important, the dock workers loved it. Their health committee promoted it, and up to 150 men lined up each day for six weeks to be tested for vision, hearing, tuberculosis, heart disease, hypertension, kidney disease, diabetes, anemia, and syphilis. Such was the description of a *San Francisco Chronicle* reporter, Harold Gilliam, in a 1951 article headlined "A Revolutionary Medical Plan Comes to the Waterfront."

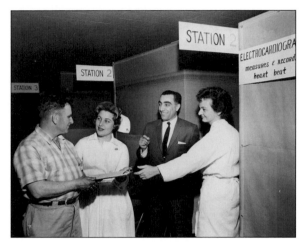

One of the thousands of ILWU workers who received multiphasic screening at the union hall, 1961.
Photo credit: International Longshoremen and Warehousemen Union.

"I feel better already," one young longshoreman told Gilliam as a union official stamped his union book to show he had completed his multiphasic. "I've worked on the docks for 40 years," said another, much older worker, "but I never dreamed I'd see something like this for longshoremen." Gilliam called it — more accurately, perhaps, than he realized — "an experiment that is making medical history."

The multiphasic screening of the port workers — because they were members of a prepaid health plan and could receive follow-up care from physicians — was the first time in American history that such medical monitoring and treatment became possible from mass testing procedures. The postwar multiphasic plan would expand to other health plan members and become a major historical development in the field of periodic health examinations in the mid-twentieth century. "The most influential experience was that of the Kaiser Permanente Health Plan in the San Francisco area," wrote Dr. Paul K.J. Han of the Division of General Internal

Medicine at the University of Pittsburgh Medical Center and Montefiore University Hospital in a 1997 *Annals of Internal Medicine* historical review of the evolution of the periodic health examination. What those working on the project in the early 1950s did not know, however, was that it also would evolve into one of the world's most important testing grounds for the use of computers in medicine.

Meanwhile, Sidney Garfield was busy on another union front. Local 770 of the Retail Clerks Union in Los Angeles had been searching independently for a health plan. Among the people its leaders consulted were Bernard B. Berkov, a medical economist, and the soon-to-be Permanente Health Plan medical director, Dr. Weinerman. The Permanente Health Plan was their choice, and Joseph T. De Silva, the union's secretary-treasurer, traveled to Oakland to talk to Garfield. Garfield explained that, as much as he wanted to expand into metropolitan Los Angeles, he did not have the necessary capital. De Silva, with gusto rivaling that of Harry Bridges, countered with an offer Garfield could hardly refuse — and one that overcame Henry Kaiser's initial resistance to further expansion into Los Angeles. With close to 30,000 union members, De Silva offered three months health plan membership dues in advance. Garfield and his southern California colleague, Ray Kay, finally could fulfill their dream of a prepaid group medical practice in Los Angeles proper. Thus, Garfield shepherded the medical care program into Los Angeles and Ray Kay, in 1953, became the founding medical director of the Southern California Permanente Medical Group.

The rapid growth of union membership over the next few years pushed enrollment toward the half million mark on the West Coast. The challenge now was having enough hospital beds, which sent Garfield literally back to his drawing board. His so-called "dream hospitals" that would open over the next few years would draw national and international acclaim. However, one of them, coupled with his increasingly complex relationship with Henry Kaiser, would lead to his fall from grace as head of the Permanente Foundation Health Plan and Hospitals, and ultimately from the medical group that had started it all.

❧ Chapter 10 ❧

Toward Tahoe: Crises and Crossroads

A poignant personal and professional bond developed between Henry J. Kaiser and Sidney Garfield as the two men, so different in temperament, background, age, and competencies, went about bringing Garfield's vision to reality. They protected the program from the critics. They ensured its sustainability. But for Garfield, the relationship, which paid great dividends, also extracted great costs.

In the early 1950s, as Garfield partnered with some of California's most prominent architects to design a series of imaginative, innovative, and efficient new hospitals, his closeness to Kaiser brought him international acclaim. It likewise undermined and toppled him as the leader of the health plan and hospital system he had created in partnership with Kaiser. In the course of a tumultuous first half of the 1950s, the Permanente name was changed to Kaiser, internal conflicts raged as the former Sidney Garfield and Associates doctors squared off against the Kaiser managers, and the whole enterprise came perilously close to implosion.

Garfield, largely as a result of unintended consequences, was caught squarely in the middle of all the tumult, between the colleagues and physicians to whom he had given his medical practice, on one side, and on the other the powerful patron,

Henry Kaiser, whose moral and financial support and genius for building things had made it all possible.

As the co-founders of the medical care program, Garfield and Kaiser already had a close relationship. Garfield had even become the Kaiser family's personal medical advisor. This evolved into a particularly close relationship starting in 1944 when Henry and Bess's younger son, Henry Jr., then 27, began to experience muscle weakness. At the time, he was running Kaiser-operated artillery shell plants in Denver, Colorado, and Fontana, California. He traveled to Oakland, where he was examined by Cecil Cutting, chief of staff of both the Oakland and Richmond hospitals. The news was bad, and Cutting had to break it to Henry and Bess: Henry Jr. had multiple sclerosis. Exhibiting his father's characteristic style, Henry Jr. refused to submit to a program of rest, undertaking instead an intense regimen of physical therapy while continuing his full work schedule.

His father, meanwhile, searched for any treatment that might offer hope: a bright ray arrived courtesy of his old journalist friend, Paul de Kruif, who in February 1946 published an article in *Reader's Digest* entitled "Many Will Rise and Walk." It described the work of Dr. Herman Kabat, a Washington, D.C., neurophysiologist and clinical neurologist who appeared to be getting dramatic improvements in multiple sclerosis patients using new methods of physical therapy as well as the drug prostigmine, which had been used to help people with a muscle weakening disease, myasthenia gravis. Kaiser Sr. asked Garfield if he would go to Washington and check out Kabat's work firsthand.

Garfield did and was impressed. "He had people walking who hadn't walked for years," recalled Garfield, who immediately put Henry Jr. under the care of Kabat and his nurse Margaret "Maggie" Knott. Garfield then sent several Permanente physicians to spend six months with Kabat, whom he ultimately decided to hire and bring to California. Thus was born the Kabat-Kaiser Research Institute, which evolved into the Kaiser Foundation Rehabilitation Center, a world-class rehabilitation medicine program in Vallejo, California, that today is Kaiser Permanente's

Center of Excellence for Culturally Competent Care for members with disabilities. (Henry Jr. died in 1961 at age 44, having maintained a busy and active career that included spearheading Kaiser Permanente's first forays into public relations.)

Garfield's growing emotional bond with Kaiser Sr. intensified still further when Bess Kaiser, who had been suffering for years with chronic high blood pressure, began to grow weaker with the added complication of progressive kidney failure. Although Garfield knew her condition was probably terminal, he sent cardiology and renal disease specialists in search of the latest treatments during the final months of her life.

At Garfield's request, Dr. Cutting, the future executive director of The Permanente Medical Group, took a leave of absence from his surgical duties at the Oakland hospital and actually moved into the Kaisers' penthouse overlooking Lake Merritt in downtown Oakland to care for Bess.

Garfield also asked a nurse at the Permanente Hospital, Alyce Chester, to move in to provide nursing care for Mrs. Kaiser. Described by those who knew her as a brilliant nurse, Chester had joined the staff during the war years. She was an at-

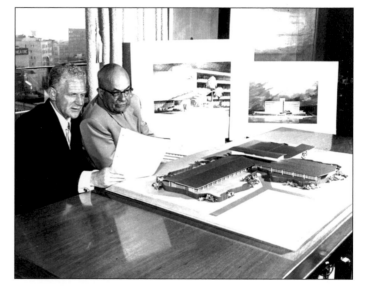

In 1952, Sidney Garfield and Henry Kaiser review a model of the controversial Walnut Creek hospital and renderings of the Los Angeles and San Francisco hospitals.

tractive woman, divorced, and the mother of a young son, Michael. Garfield had mentored her and, impressed with her abilities, made her a part of his executive team and increasingly came to rely on her. However, his decision to have Chester care for Bess would prove far more fateful than he could have imagined.

With Mrs. Kaiser's needs attended to with expert 24-hour care, Garfield was busy on another front. To handle the medical needs of the burgeoning number of health plan members in California, he made plans for the expansion of the Oakland and Vallejo hospitals and construction of two new, 210-bed hospitals — the first in Los

Angeles on Sunset Boulevard near downtown, while the second, a virtual duplicate of the first, was built on Geary Boulevard in San Francisco. Each would have adjacent, 12,000-square-foot medical office buildings. They were highly innovative designs and came to be widely referred to as "dream hospitals," due to their generally airy and spacious accommodations and patient-centric creature comforts.

Behind the scenes, however, big problems brewed. On March 15, 1951, Bess Kaiser, who was a beloved figure across the medical care program and all of Kaiser Industries, died. Within a month, the widowed Kaiser, 68, shocked everyone by announcing he would marry Alyce Chester, 34. The two had grown close during Bess's illness. The marriage was strongly opposed by Kaiser's two sons, who were Chester's age, along with most of Kaiser's executives. Garfield, however, supported Kaiser, at least in part because he knew Kaiser dreaded living alone. Also, he may have known or suspected that Bess Kaiser had blessed the union because she understood so well Kaiser's need for an intimate companion.

Now the Garfield-Kaiser relationship took another, more complicated twist when Alyce Kaiser's equally pretty younger sister, Helen Chester Peterson, divorced within the year and Garfield fell in love with her. Henry Kaiser was thrilled, even playing the Cupid role, actively encouraging their marriage. The wedding came as a surprise to even Garfield's closest friends. Indeed, he was living with one of his oldest physician friends at the time, Cecil Cutting, who knew nothing of wedding plans until a midnight phone call after he returned home from a long day of salmon fishing off the San Francisco coast. "Mr. Kaiser wants you down at the airport right away," the unidentified caller announced. "Sid's getting married." Garfield then came on the line. He asked Cutting to bring a suit and a clean shirt to the Oakland Airport. An hour later, Cutting and his wife, Millie, Dr. and Mrs. Wallace Neighbor, Henry and Alyce Kaiser joined Garfield and his bride to fly to Reno on Kaiser's private DC-3 for a city hall ceremony.

The newlyweds moved into a house next door to a new mansion Kaiser had just built in Lafayette, a wealthy bedroom community in Contra Costa County 10 miles east of Oakland. Sidney Garfield and Henry Kaiser now were co-founders of the medical care program, close-friends-turned-brothers-in-law, and next-door neighbors. Sisters Alyce and Helen also were very close, and the two couples spent most evenings together over cocktails, dinner, and conversation.

However noble his interest may have been, Kaiser now was taking a larger and more problematic role in the medical care program, at the expense of Garfield's own influence and leadership. While the attack from the medical society in Alameda County ended with endorsement of the program, concerns over lay control of medical practice at the national level of the medical establishment were as strong as ever. Whereas there had always been a gentlemen's agreement that physicians were in control of the Permanente medical program, Kaiser, the layman, was continually testing the dividing line, even when in 1948 he threatened to sue the Alameda County Medical Association on behalf of his beleaguered colleague, Sidney Garfield.

Symptomatic of this tendency was Kaiser's planning for a third new "dream hospital" to be located in Walnut Creek, a then rural town a few miles east of the Kaiser/Garfield compound in Lafayette. Kaiser, in Garfield's words, saw this project as "an interesting job for his (Kaiser's) new wife — to give her an interest outside of social interests." Garfield, apparently caught up in the early stages of the design discussions, which he loved, offered no opposition. Indeed, one evening after dinner the two couples began moving furniture around Kaiser's living room and dining room, using it to kick around ideas for how they would mock up a design for the hospital.

However, no one consulted the Permanente Medical Groups in California about the Walnut Creek plans, nor had there been any discussion of even a need for another hospital while planning was proceeding for hospitals to meet the needs of 150,000 members in Los Angeles and San Francisco, compared with a mere 5,000 members living in the Walnut Creek area. Thus, the Permanente physicians in Oakland, rightly proud of the system they had built with Garfield, had to be especially stunned when Kaiser unilaterally announced plans for the Walnut Creek hospital. To make matters worse, he boasted that Walnut Creek would be a medical showcase and would be open to use by local fee-for-service physicians, not just the prepaid Permanente Medical Group based in Oakland. And while construction costs were closely controlled in building the Los Angeles and San Francisco hospitals, money seemed to be no object for the Walnut Creek hospital, which Garfield personally designed. In a typical gesture, Kaiser himself drove a bulldozer as site preparation started. The beautiful and genuinely innovative hospital opened six months before either Los Angeles or San Francisco. And to add insult to injury, it became the poster child of cutting-edge hospitals, with a major photo and text spread in *Look Magazine*. It also was the subject of a *Universal-International* newsreel story, "Dream Hospital: It's the Last Word in Modern Design," on movie screens across the U.S.

The Walnut Creek hospital — while it proved very successful in the long view of history — became one of several symbols of Henry Kaiser's intrusion into medical matters after his second marriage and one of multiple triggers for the near death of the entire organization. One of the other issues, however, added a less substantive, if more symbolically potent, irritant to the raw and prickly feelings that Kaiser was causing among the Oakland doctors. This was the decision to replace the name Permanente with Kaiser, based on the reasonable argument that the Kaiser name was well-known and easier to pronounce than Permanente. Garfield, again, went along with "the Boss," but only as far as the name change applied to the health plan and hospitals. Like the rest of the Permanente doctors, he strongly opposed changing the medical group name to the Kaiser Medical Group. They, too, had a compelling reason. With continuing claims by the local medical societies that the Permanente physicians were under the control of Henry Kaiser, a layman, the name change would only have served to further reinforce the notion that they were "Kaiser doctors."

It fell to Garfield's old friend, Ray Kay, head of the southern California Permanente group, to break the news of the doctors' opposition to Kaiser, because Garfield refused to do it. Kay had taken the train to Oakland for other business, and Garfield picked him up at the station.

"Ray," Garfield told him, "you're going to have to talk to Mr. Kaiser about the name."

"Oh, my lord," Kay muttered, filled with dread.

When they got to Kaiser's office, they gathered around a huge conference table. At one end sat Kaiser, at the other Garfield. In the middle, across from one another, were Kay and key Kaiser executive Eugene Trefethen.

"Ray," Trefethen began, "tell Mr. Kaiser why you think the medical group shouldn't use the Kaiser name."

Kay told Kaiser that the medical group had no grounds for opposing him on the renaming of the health plan and hospitals, but that the name "Kaiser Medical Group … would just hurt us even more … It would give truth to that lie that we were just (Kaiser doctors)."

Trefethen tactfully broke the silence: "Well, Mr. Kaiser, I think there's some merit in what Ray is saying."

"Of course, of course," Kaiser responded. Then he sulked, "I don't want them to use my name. I wouldn't let them use my name."

It was, Kay recollected, "just as if we'd taken candy away from him."

The rift between the physicians and "the Kaiser people," a term which tended to uncomfortably include Garfield, was growing and came to a head at a tense three-day meeting — later named the "Tahoe Conference" — at Kaiser's scenic mountain estate near Homewood on the shore of Lake Tahoe in 1955 (later made famous by Hollywood as a key setting in the second of the "Godfather" movie series). Before that meeting could settle matters, Garfield's own ambiguous status as a Kaiser loyalist dedicated to Permanente independence had to be resolved.

That bitter resolution came the night before the convening of the Tahoe Conference, where Garfield was expected to represent the positions of the medical groups. By this time, Garfield had already made Alyce Kaiser the director of operations of the new medical center. But Henry wanted something more. The "can-do" industrialist was impatient with the checks and balances the physicians imposed on his freedom to act. He proposed a solution. "I think we ought to have a separate partnership over in Walnut Creek," he declared to Garfield. "We want to pay our [Walnut Creek] doctors more money and we want to build up this [partnership] to be the finest organization in the country."

Garfield argued that a separate medical partnership in northern California would not work, but in the end he agreed to try to sell the Oakland physicians on the idea.

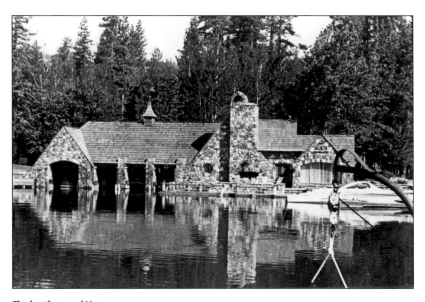

The boathouse of Henry Kaiser's fabled "Fleur de Lac" estate at Lake Tahoe, the only building that survives to this day. It was here that Henry Kaiser and his executives and Permanente leaders negotiated the Tahoe agreement, the basis for the enduring Kaiser Permanente partnership.

As time passed, Kaiser grew more and more irritated that he could not get the control he wanted, and he blamed his brother-in-law. As Garfield later recalled it: "He finally decided that I was a particular part of that problem. I couldn't get the job done and he said I promised him I would get it done. He suggested that possibly they put somebody else in my place, and I said, 'Well, that's fine with me, if you want to do that.'"

Kaiser and Garfield met in Kaiser's home office in Lafayette. Kaiser told him he had to step down as medical director of the health plan and hospitals. They argued, and Kaiser finally said, "Sidney, whether you want it or not, it's got to be done." Garfield finally countered that he would step aside only if the physicians attending the Tahoe meeting from Oakland, Los Angeles, and Portland agreed, calculating they would not. He was wrong. By then, they too had concluded that whatever his genius for innovation and his selfless dedication to building the original Permanente program, he was no longer the right man to lead a very large and complex organization that needed a firm physician's hand at the helm.

Lambreth Hancock, who was executive assistant to Kaiser and an eyewitness to the negotiations at Tahoe, described the sessions as "stomach-wrenching." But given Garfield's compromised position, caught in the middle as he was between Kaiser and the doctors, the action was necessary in the view of George Link, an attorney and member of the Kaiser management group at the Tahoe meeting: "Management had to be clarified, and as long as Sidney was there, it was going to be a mishmash."

The Tahoe summit was painful on all sides. Yet it shaped a new management structure that still serves as a model in the annals of American medicine. And it illuminated the character of the parties on all sides as they grappled with anguishing issues and came away the better for it. In the end, Kaiser ceded control of medical matters to the physicians. The doctors recognized the importance of having trained business professionals running the health plan and hospital organizations, with proper physician input. The health plan and hospitals would retain the name Kaiser, while the physicians would keep the name Permanente, thus leading to the lasting organizational name of Kaiser Permanente.

Of the demotion of Sidney Garfield, Hancock later said, "Once the decision was made, there were no grudges held, and he and Mr. Kaiser and everybody else were still just as close as they ever were." Added Link, "All of these people — and I say all of them, and I believe all of them — were men of good will. They wanted to make this thing work. There were … hard meetings where people got angry with each other. But they really wanted to make it work."

History has judged them all well. Ultimately, they wanted to hold to the historic mission of the medical care program — affordable, quality health care services to improve the health of its members and the communities it served. To achieve this, the Tahoe Conference created shared management through separate, but closely cooperating partnership organizations. Kaiser Foundation Health Plans in each geographic region would be nonprofit, public benefit corporations that would contract with individuals and groups to arrange for comprehensive medical and hospital services. Kaiser Foundation Hospitals, as nonprofit, public benefit corporations, would own and operate community hospitals and outpatient facilities or arrange contracts for hospital services. They would sponsor charitable, educational and research activities. The Permanente Medical Groups, through a mutually exclusive contract with the health plan, would assume full responsibility for providing and arranging necessary medical care for the health plan members in each region. The mutually exclusive nature of the relationship meant that every entity depended on every other entity for its success, a fact that has always argued forcefully for the integration and alignment of financial and strategic goals.

The first full history of the events at Tahoe was written two decades later by Greer Williams, an assistant professor at Tufts University School of Medicine. He called the settlements reached at Tahoe the "Tahoe Agreement" — a term which acquired almost mythic status among subsequent Kaiser Permanente generations. He also referred to it as "the Tahoe commitment" and concluded it was not merely a watershed for Kaiser Permanente, but also a milestone in American medical history:

"The Tahoe commitment ... may well be regarded as one of the most significant moments in the history of medical care organizations," he wrote. "If the observer had to single out one characteristic more essential to the success of the Kaiser Permanente health plan than all others, it would be the capacity of the organization that has evolved to project the doctor-patient relationship through a marriage of medicine and management in the service of millions of patients."

Despite the historic outcome at Tahoe, Sidney Garfield emerged from these events at probably the lowest point of his life. In the months leading up to Tahoe he had been energetically tackling the design and construction of multiple hospitals, dealing with the explosive growth in health plan membership, fighting periodic flares of criticism from the medical establishment, and getting accustomed to married life. He had also recently faced the grief that came with the deaths of his elderly parents, Isaac and Bertha, one not long after the other. Now, Garfield left Tahoe stripped of his leadership over the organizations he had created.

Chapter 11

After Tahoe:
Pursuing New Frontiers

Sidney Garfield's loss of his leadership positions in 1955 could never strip him of his prominence as founding physician. Whereas some saw him as marginalized, or "defrocked," most people who mattered, both within and outside the organization, continued to seek and value his judgment on issues of strategic importance, if not operational ones. He was playing a new role as vice president for facilities design, and later joined the boards of directors of Kaiser Foundation Health Plan and Kaiser Foundation Hospitals. And only months after the meeting at Tahoe, it was Sidney Garfield who was testifying on emerging health insurance policy matters before the California Legislature. He was the one to whom people looked to explain the medical care program that was rapidly growing into the largest, not-for-profit health care delivery system in the United States. As George Link said, "There were no grudges held."

Garfield — acting a lot like he did when his immigrant parents demanded he become a physician rather than an architect or engineer — played the cards he was dealt. He went on to do outstanding things over the next few decades in hospital design, trying to improve efficiency while always focusing on the needs of patients and hospital staff. More than two decades before the personal computer was introduced, he was thinking about how computers could be adapted to medicine.

When his integrated, prevention-oriented, group practice delivery system came to be viewed as a national model for improved quality and efficiency in the 1970s, he acknowledged the praise and then argued that the delivery system he created had become the equivalent of a "horse and buggy" in need of a fundamental revision. Out of this thinking came "The Delivery of Medical Care," published in *Scientific American* in April 1970 (Appendix 5), the most important paper of his career. It laid the foundation for the modern Kaiser Permanente.

Garfield's quest was to do all that he could to make Kaiser Permanente a "total health" organization, one which was truly "a health plan, not a sick plan." So when Sidney Garfield later reflected on his life after Tahoe, he was philosophical. "What has grown out of (Tahoe) is a stronger organization, a stronger realization on both the Kaiser and the physicians' side of the importance of working together … So that was good … Something good comes out of everything."

Each new phase of Garfield's life after the Tahoe meeting built on the previous one, starting with hospital design. The wartime operating suite at Vancouver, with its design of "clean" and "dirty" corridors and the supervisor in the middle, was his "first important breakthrough in hospital design," by his own calculation. Over the next three decades, he modified that innovation, which came to be called "the central workspace-peripheral corridor concept," incorporating it successively into radiological suites, labor and delivery, first aid stations, emergency departments, intensive care units, coronary units, nursing units, and patient wings.

Garfield's design ideas were strongly influenced by those of Louis Sullivan, the famed Chicago architect and "father of modernism" who coined the term "form follows function." Indeed, in writing about trying to design the ideal nursing unit in the *Journal of the American Hospital Association* in 1971, Garfield opened by quoting Sullivan's famous 1896 line: "Over all the coursing sun, form follows function, and that is the law."

"Concern with efficient design of its hospitals has been inherent in the evolution of the Kaiser Foundation Health Plan and Hospitals," Garfield explained. "Because … [it is] committed to providing the best possible care at the most reasonable cost, and because it must build and pay for its facilities without benefit of subsidy or philanthropy, it has been vital to its existence and development that planning should efficiently link form and function."

The Walnut Creek Kaiser Foundation Hospital, despite the controversy it stirred and the political costs for Garfield, was a crowning achievement from the standpoint of innovation, efficiency, and design, as were the San Francisco and Los Angeles hospitals that contained similar features. "A new day has dawned, where more brains will go into the design and architecture of a hospital," Dr. Walter C. Alvarez, a famed Mayo Clinic internist, said of Garfield's designs in a nationally broadcast radio interview in 1953. Citing pneumatic tube systems that improved delivery of patient records, Ed Herlihy, narrator of the "Dream Hospital" newsreel about the Walnut Creek design commented, "The patient's record reaches the doctor before he [the patient] does." In Los Angeles, newscaster Chet Huntley, then with the American Broadcasting Company, declared in a broadcast on June 24, 1953: "The use of labor-saving devices, the use of light (both natural and artificial), the furnishings, the gadgets, the décor and the personnel are all combined to make the new Kaiser Foundation Hospital something special."

Trained as neither architect nor engineer, Garfield had to work closely with noted architects to develop and implement the design features he thought up. They were impressed with his ideas and learned from him. The corridor system evolved as he called for three corridors for the entire hospital, each for its own traffic. Physicians, nurses, and other staff would use the central service corridor to take care of patients, whose rooms were on each side. Here, in close proximity to patients, were located decentralized nursing stations, supply cupboards, medical records units, and some of the nation's first microwave ovens, for serving hot meals to patients. Two more corridors provided walkways outside patients' rooms on both sides of the hospital building. Visitors would arrive through these corridors, accessing patient rooms through sliding glass doors, so as not to interfere with hospital personnel.

In March 1954, the Walnut Creek facility was named "Hospital of the Month" by *Modern Hospital Magazine*. In the accompanying article, Clarence Mayhew, the San Francisco-based architect for the Walnut Creek hospital, commented about how much he had learned from Garfield. "The idea of a 'Nursing and Utility Corridor' is the basic plan pattern around which the entire hospital is designed," he wrote. "This new concept resulted from a never-ending search for ways to improve patient care by increasing the efficiency of the nurse."

"In other words," the architect continued, "the patient's charts, medicines, treatment materials, equipment and utilities which the nurse uses in her work [were generally] too far removed from the patient. The solution was to locate the patient's charts, medicines, treatment materials, equipment and utilities along the central corridor … The central corridor becomes work space and the nurses'

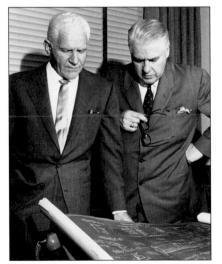

Sidney Garfield and Clarence Mayhew, architect of the Walnut Creek hospital and an ardent admirer of Garfield's hospital designs, 1962.

station, utility equipment, drugs, X-rays, treatment materials, instruments, linens, charts and so on for each patient can be kept in this workspace just behind the patient's room."

The end result, Mayhew said, was that the design saved "six out of every seven steps" for the nurse. The nurses were closer to the patients and could more efficiently answer their calls. Better observation of patients was possible. Medication was close by. The physician could enter the patient's room with the entire record in hand.

The biggest design hit at Garfield's 1950s-era hospitals was the so-called "Baby in the Drawer," a concept adapted from an experiment at Yale University's medical school hospital. It was a prime example of the kind of innovation Garfield sought. It played a major role in reducing nursing steps, was cost-effective because it increased efficiency, and research showed it improved mother-baby bonding. Garfield arranged that each mother's room would be adjacent to the nursery, with the baby in a bassinet set in an ordinary metal file drawer built into the wall separating the mother's room and the nursery. The mother could roll the mobile bassinet to her bedside to feed or hold her baby, and then return the infant to the nursery. This allowed a newborn to be adjacent to its mother while also being under the direct supervision of the medical staff. A simple light signal would tell the nurse whether a baby was in the nursery or in its mother's room. This functional design was based on Garfield's belief that the earliest contacts between mother and baby should be encouraged. Subsequent studies showed that large numbers of mothers chose to breast-feed as a result of the system.

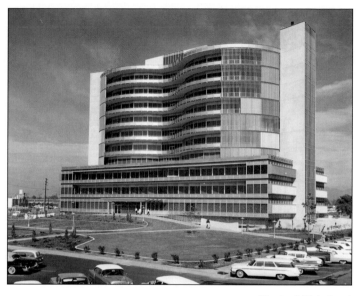

The Garfield-designed Panorama City, California hospital on opening day, 1962.

In addition, every patient room had no more than two beds. Ambulatory patients could go to the top floor of each of the hospitals, which was designed to create a hotel-like ambiance. They also could choose to go to a dining room for buffet meals, could sleep late in the morning, and could avail themselves of planned recreation and social activities.

Garfield's avocation was now his vocation. His appetite had been whetted with the surgical suite at Vancouver in 1943, which hospital design experts from all over the country came to view. When he rebuilt the old, abandoned hospital in Oakland for wartime use and expanded it, an architectural reviewer raved about its modern features: "… if you ever are ill enough to need hospitalization, you will want to get to the Permanente Foundation Hospital in Oakland, no matter where you are," wrote architect Mark Daniels. After San Francisco, Los Angeles, and

89

Walnut Creek, Garfield oversaw the design of new hospitals in Honolulu (1958), Portland (1959), Panorama City (1962), and Santa Clara (1964), the latter two in California. Each design improved upon the previous one. Panorama City was an experiment that adapted his Honolulu hospital into a circular building design. Overall, that did not work out but the circular nursing stations in the building proved effective and were put into the Santa Clara hospital, which gravitated back to a rectangular building design.

In the process of this decade-long expansion in the number of Kaiser hospitals, a collaborative process also evolved that incorporated suggestions from the physicians, nurses, and staff who had to use the facility. "When the plans for a new hospital are being worked on," Garfield explained, "copies are sent to the regional administrators and physicians in the area served by the hospital and to those in other areas for advice and suggestions. The advice, suggestions and objections, if any, are sifted and weighed, and compromises are reached before the plans are put into final form. This procedure is preferable to the autocratic way of saying: 'This is how it's going to be.'" It was not always an easy process, compared with a top-down one. "The democratic approach can be a little 'traumatic,'" Garfield once acknowledged.

By 1960, Garfield, now 54, had added a complex system of hospitals in four states to his ever expanding delivery system, and he was beginning to look beyond the drawing board for new challenges. As correspondent Jane Barton wrote in *Modern Hospital* magazine in 1962, "While Dr. Garfield is busily planning new hospitals he would really like nothing better than to put himself out of business as a hospital planner. This will come when preventive medicine, which he considers the best medicine of all, can be developed to a point [at which] the demand for hospital beds is replaced by a demand for the kind of care that will keep people out of bed." Besides this growing concern for wellness care and what he termed "total health," Garfield was beginning to sense that the essential key to improvements in both wellness and sick care had more to do with the information that could be contained and conveyed in the bits and bytes of computer data than in the bricks and mortar of his hospitals. Those pneumatic tubes that whisked paper-based patient charts throughout the new hospitals were already looking a bit archaic.

When Garfield addressed a Kaiser management conference at Monterey, California, in May 1960 (Appendix 3), he talked about the new hospitals under construction, innovations in food service, new methods of distribution of supplies, new manufacturing methods of IV solution, modern ultrasonic laundry equipment, and other facility-related innovations. Then he changed the subject to propose what he called "a more important, new concept."

"I want to throw this idea on the table for your consideration," he declared. "Please accept it in the spirit it is given. It is a controversial idea, but please keep an open mind." With that, he proposed Kaiser Permanente become a vanguard on the new frontier of medical computing.

"It's really time for us to revitalize our plan," he argued. "I suggest a radical new idea — that we stop building hospitals and clinics for sick people. Let's concentrate on a brand new type of facility — a new first in the world. Let us conceive a building for health — designed, streamlined, and geared to serve our healthy members."

Garfield said he envisioned a time when a medical history of a new health plan member would be fed into a computer — using the then cutting-edge technology of punch cards and IBM mainframes. At each visit thereafter, he explained, "further data would be taken … and fed into this record. This would … develop records never before available …" Eventually, he continued, health care facilities would all feature high-tech centers focused on prevention and health maintenance, "where every conceivable laboratory, X-ray, EKG, and other tests could be run by such advanced new equipment …" To this, he said, add a health education program, well-baby clinics, prenatal clinics, teenage clinics, and a place for routine vaccinations and immunizations.

Garfield anticipated that the greatest fear his ideas would trigger would be that computers would depersonalize the all-important, and often intimate and trusting, doctor-patient relationship. Preempting such concerns, he argued that just the opposite would be true. The physician would have greater access to more medical information about every patient. "This 'doctor-patient relationship' becomes important when the patient becomes sick, and the available records, the education of the member about his plan, and other features might give the physician a much sounder base for better doctor-patient relations than he has today," he argued.

Already a true believer in this "radical new idea," Garfield said he envisioned his wellness-oriented "health plan" as something that could lead American health policy in new directions, just as his original prepaid group practice delivery system had established a national precedent. "It is interesting to conjecture and dream of the impact of this …" he said. "First, it might advance us from the horse and buggy stage to 20 years ahead of our times again. It certainly would give our health plan … a true preventive program — something dreamed about by all plans but never accomplished before … It could sweep the country."

Dr. John G. Smillie, who recorded notes from discussion groups at the two-day meeting, commented that health plan leaders and physicians who reflected on Garfield's proposal thought it "had exciting merit" and "should be studied from many angles, designed and redesigned." Reflecting the embedded core value that new ideas should be tested scientifically and advanced when they showed demonstrated value, Smillie added, "The group endorsed any feasible move in this direction, but with open eyes." Perhaps, it was suggested, the U.S. Public Health Service could finance the work in whole or part.

One thing was certain. No one at that Monterey meeting viewed Sidney Garfield as a defrocked former leader. He was still Kaiser Permanente's chief source of vision and inspiration.

❧ Chapter 12 ❧

The Best Is Yet to Come

"Personally," Sidney Garfield once said, "I am more interested in the future than the past." Yet he clearly understood the past, and often drew lessons from history. Perhaps it was that combination of the historical perspective and the focus on what was to come that sustained his lifelong ability to march past adversity and into the future. Having been moved to the fringe of the organizations that he co-founded with Henry Kaiser, the "fringe" for Garfield — no matter the personal injury he undoubtedly felt — gave him

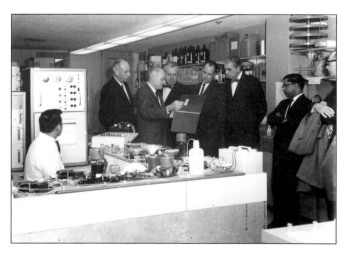

Morris Collen with Cecil Cutting lead a delegation of national public health leaders on a tour of the Automated Multiphasic Health Testing facility in 1966. Among them were Congressman John Fogarty, who subsequently introduced legislation to replicate Collen's work around the country.

the opportunity to explore the far horizons of medicine. As his younger colleague and Permanente historian Dr. John Smillie would later write, "Sidney Garfield, after all, had a way of always operating on the cutting edge of the future."

Garfield, as ever, remained a fount of radical new ideas, never satisfied with what was. In the 1960s, he grew frustrated that Kaiser Permanente had not evolved further than it had. He still wanted to create what he started to call a "total health" delivery system, one that focused on the healthy patients as well as the sick. He wanted his true "health plan," not a "sick plan." In this context, he became more and more fascinated with nascent ideas about medicine and computer electronics that were beginning to be talked about in scientific circles.

Garfield shared his frustrations with his old friend Cecil Cutting, by then executive director of The Permanente Medical Group. Cutting, a quiet and steady leader, grounded in wisdom and patience, shared the vision of new frontiers in medicine, and together they looked for someone with the right skills to explore these ideas about computers and medicine. They didn't have to look far, for there was only one choice: Dr. Morris F. Collen. Having always wanted a career in academic medicine, Collen's dream had been short-circuited by World War II. However, he had nevertheless vigorously engaged in the medical care program's research projects since World War II as editor of the *Permanente Foundation Medical Bulletin,* a quarterly research journal, and as author of numerous, groundbreaking, published research studies. He had also initiated and led an ambitious health screening and early detection program for Kaiser Permanente adult members known as Multiphasic Health Testing. As for computer knowledge, he had a unique qualification: before he decided to go to medical school, Collen had earned his bachelor's degree in electrical engineering at the University of Minnesota in 1934. When he decided to go to medical school, he met with Dr. Elias Lyon, Dean of Minnesota's School of Medicine, who burst into laughter when Collen said he wanted to enroll. "What's the matter?" Dr. Lyon asked. "Can't they find jobs for you engineers?" When Collen explained that he wanted to apply his training in electro-organic chemistry, Lyon understood he was serious. With some additional coursework in zoology, Collen gained admission.

Garfield explained that he believed the medical care program needed to make use of computers. Would Collen attend an upcoming international meeting on the topic and advise Cutting and himself? "Well," Collen later recalled, "I came back and advised them that Dr. Garfield was correct …"

Such was the beginning of a long and remarkable career that would, over many decades, place Morris Collen — and Kaiser Permanente — at the forefront of the brave new world of "medical informatics," or what some today refer to as "health IT." Indeed, many years later, when the time came to establish the ultimate award in the field, it would be named the Morris F. Collen Award of Excellence, and Collen himself was the first recipient.

Work on adapting the computer to the Permanente practice style (what today is called Permanente Medicine) — and on building the "total health" organization that Garfield envisioned — began in earnest in 1961. As Cutting reported to the Executive Committee of The Permanente Medical Group in September of that year, Collen, in a new role, would explore and develop the "health" aspects of medical care activities, as proposed by Garfield at the Monterey Conference (Appendix 3). The work would proceed in multiple directions — expansion and modernization of the Multiphasic Health Testing program, including establishment of a pediatric screening program; expansion of the use of paramedical personnel, where appropriate, to free up physicians' time; the use of "all possible electronic aids in diagnostic work and treatment"; the creation of a special program for the growing number of geriatric problems; improved methods of recording and tabulating patient clinical information; and

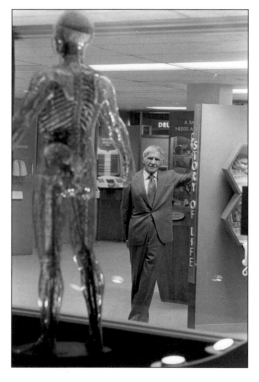

Sidney Garfield with the Transparent Man, purchased from the Expo '67 in Montreal, as an experimental tool in Kaiser Permanente's groundbreaking Health Education Center.

increased emphasis throughout the program on preventive medicine. With that, the Executive Committee approved Collen's appointment as founding director of a new department called Medical Methods Research, later renamed the Division of Research, in Oakland, California.

The fundamental question regarding the use of computers, was whether they could be adapted to medicine on a mass scale. Collen had been working on multiphasic screening for a decade at that point. The program involved a series of basic, repetitive tests, and physical examinations that concluded with manually recording voluminous amounts of medical data about each and every patient. Though the clinicians who conducted the exams knew the work was medically important, they found it tedious and boring. Thus, it seemed to Collen to be the perfect first experiment in computerizing medical data, and the idea of "*automated* Multiphasic Health Testing" was born. The U.S. Public Health Service, which had been suggested as a funding source at the Monterey Conference, provided a $300,000 grant in 1961 to help build an Automated Multiphasic Health Testing (AMHT) facility in Oakland. This allowed 35,000 patients to go through the program in the first year — a half-million people by the end of a decade.

David Perlman, a distinguished science journalist, described the process to the public in lay terms a few years later in the *San Francisco Chronicle*. "Patients," he wrote after touring the program, "undergo what must be the most exhaustive 'routine' checkup in the world."

"For three hours or more," he explained, "they are photographed, X-rayed, questioned, and cardiographed. They answer hundreds of medical and psychological queries on IBM cards. Their blood and urine are sampled; their eyes and hearing are tested; their tendons are squeezed; their lung capacity is probed; their pulse and blood pressure are registered. And all the while a great IBM 1440 computer system is swiftly storing the data in its capacious magnetic memory, processing the facts and figures, and preparing its automated reports, patient by patient … By the time a Kaiser patient has finished his checkup, clad briefly in a disposable paper gown and grasping a clipboard stuffed with IBM cards and question sheets, the Kaiser machines know far more about him than he does himself. But most important, the machines will be able to furnish the patient's doctor with an enormously complete sum-mary of everything the tests show, so that the patient's face-to-face physical examination can be truly productive."

Over the next decade and a half, the vast amount of clinical data on these Kaiser Permanente members enabled the research team that Collen gathered to produce more than 500 research papers published in more than 75 medical journals.

In the first few years, however, there were, certainly, skeptics about the value of computerization among Collen's fellow Permanente physicians. Garfield addressed the skepticism in 1965 with a steady eye on the future. "As physicians, you can benefit in many ways," he told doctors at an educational conference titled Medicine of the Future. "With computerized history and findings available from basic evaluations, you will know more about your patients than you do today — you will be able to serve them better and treat them more rationally." He laid out a vision of computerized medical information being linked with health education programs and teams made up of physicians and ancillary health professionals organized into a complete system of primary care to serve both the healthy and sick patient. For conservatives who wanted to wait for more results from, or even completion of, Collen's research before proceeding, Garfield declared, "I don't think we can afford to wait. Time is short … We should get into it and if the things we do don't work, try others. Trial and error is good." He boldly challenged them: "Your opportunity is that you can make history by leading the way. You have nothing to lose and everything to gain."

The very next year Kaiser Permanente exploded onto the national stage as buzz about the results of the research spread throughout the medical profession, and even among politicians. Dr. Ernest Saward, the Medical Director of the Northwest Permanente Medical Group in Portland, Oregon, and a man who traveled the globe, told Garfield that all over the world "people know more about Permanente and Kaiser Foundation because of Dr. Collen's work" than for any other reason. That was precursory to what happened next in the United States — a vigorous public health debate.

Among the curious onlookers of the multiphasic program were prominent health reformers in Congress and the U.S. Public Health Service. In January 1966, a distinguished group of federal and state officials, including Democratic Congressman John Fogarty of Rhode Island and officials of the U.S. Public Health Service, descended on Oakland. They were interested in preventive medicine and the use of computers in both medical research and medical care. Other delegations followed, including one led by then Surgeon General William Stewart, M.D., who toured the Automated Multiphasic Health Testing program.

Meanwhile, Congressman Fogarty had been so impressed by what he had learned that he introduced legislation to create regional and community centers to screen patients for disease, citing the work of Collen and his team as a pilot for what he had in mind. That August, Senator Maurine Neuberger, a Democrat from Oregon, held hearings as chair of a Special Committee on Aging. Kaiser Permanente was center stage with testimony from Collen, as well as others, who pointed to his work as an example of what was becoming possible. A new word — Preventicare — was coined in the process. "Witness after witness," reported *Time* magazine, "testified that the most promising approach to Preventicare is called 'multiphasic testing,' a program that the California-based Kaiser Foundation Health Plan has been offering its members ever since 1950. The Kaiser multiphasic checkup consists of 20 computer-oriented tests given by a team of technicians, nurses, and machines." By the end of the 1970s, Collen's work had spawned close to 400 multiphasic testing programs around the world.

With the proven value of computerized clinical data provided by the Multiphasic Health Testing program, the federal Food and Drug Administration contracted with Collen's Medical Methods Research program to pilot a drug reaction monitoring system in Kaiser Permanente's San Francisco Medical Center. Data concerning some 1,200 drug prescriptions per day were entered in the system by pharmacists, enabling emergency room physicians to have virtually instant

electronic access to drug and other laboratory data on ER patients — an early
demonstration of the medical management capabilities of the electronic medical
record that was still some 40 years in the future.

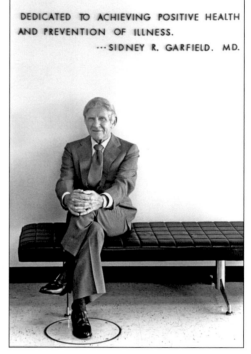

DEDICATED TO ACHIEVING POSITIVE HEALTH AND PREVENTION OF ILLNESS.
··· SIDNEY R. GARFIELD. MD.

Collen's name was now synonymous with the
birth of the new field of medical informatics, and over
the next half century — right up to the time of this
writing — he would remain at the forefront of the
field. But, however much Collen was credited with the
breakthroughs, he always maintained that the "vision"
started with "Dr. Garfield" (never referring to him by
his first name, despite their long and close relationship).
"He'd come up with all these wonderful ideas," Collen
would say, with respect and awe.

Meanwhile, the visionary Garfield was hard at work
on other projects as the fruits of Collen's work grew.
On one front, Garfield asked Collen's wife, Bobbie, a

**Sidney Garfield
in the Health
Education Center.**

registered nurse, to take on a different aspect of work — an experimental, research-
based health education center that would help both healthy and sick members play
a more active role in their own health care. Although health education programs
had long been conducted by public health agencies, this one was one of the first
such programs to be created by a private health care organization, and it broke new
ground in attitudes about health care by emphasizing the notion that patients have
a personal responsibility to maintain a healthy lifestyle. Established in Oakland
in 1969 using the nonprofit health plan's community benefit funds, the Health
Center, open to the general public, pioneered new approaches to health education
and prevention that spread across Kaiser Permanente and beyond. It included in-
person classes, multimedia recordings and films on various health topics, and even

an exhibit purchased from Expo '67 in Montreal, Canada, featuring a transparent man and a transparent woman as examples of electronic teaching machines that revealed body systems not ordinarily visible.

By the end of the 1960s, much of Garfield's vision of a new health-oriented, computer-enabled medical care system was becoming a reality. "The great promise of computers for medicine lies in making an entirely new medical care system possible," he wrote in a 1974 essay, in which he first used the term "total health care." "Such a new system is just now beginning to take form and emerge from the old."

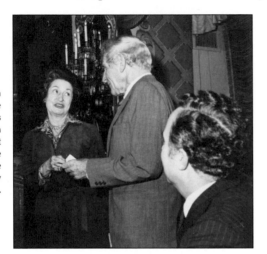

Lady Bird Johnson presenting the Lyndon Baines Johnson Foundation Award for Significant Contribution in the Field of Health Care Delivery to Sidney Garfield, 1977.

He continued: "*Health care* [emphasis in original] is a new division of medicine that does not exist in this country or any country. Its purpose is to improve health and keep people well. The system holds great promise for the provision of truly preventive care. We need no longer generalize, but instead we can instruct each individual about what he should do for optimal health on the basis of his own updated profile."

"This change from episodic crisis sick care to programmed total health care," Garfield wrote, "forces a new look at the recording and processing of medical information … Continuing total health care requires a continuing life record for each individual … The content of that life record, now made possible by computer information technology, will chart the course to be taken by each individual for optimal health."

A decade after he first discussed his vision of a new kind of total health care system, it was now time for Garfield to sum up his thinking. Putting pen to paper, he crafted what was the most important — and most cited — article of his career, "The Delivery of Medical Care," published in the April 1970 issue of

Scientific American. In it, he ambitiously called for using the computer to build the best delivery system in history: "Matching the superb technology of present day medicine with an effective delivery system can raise U.S. medical care to a level unparalleled in the world." Twenty-four years later, the article was still considered of such significance that it was republished as a Classic Article in Medical Computing in the journal *M.D. Computing.*

The solution to an outmoded delivery system built to serve the sick but not the well, he argued, was an entirely new kind of medical care organization. The computer would replace the hospital as the heart of the delivery system. The computer center would function as the central brain and help coordinate services on the basis of patients' needs — be they well or sick.

All patients, Garfield proposed, would pass through a health testing and referral service, with an automated multiphasic testing program acting as the flow regulator, in place of fee-for-service. Patients would be sorted into three categories, on the basis of their individual medical needs.

Garfield saw well and "worried well" patients being triaged to a "health care center" emphasizing wellness and offering health education, immunizations, exercise programs, psychological counseling, family planning, nutrition information, and well-baby care. Well-trained paraprofessionals, under the supervision of a physician, would serve the patients.

The second category, patients with diagnosed chronic conditions such as obesity, diabetes, hypertension, and arthritis, would be referred to a "preventive maintenance service," also staffed by paraprofessionals under physician supervision. There, they would receive routine care management, careful monitoring of their conditions, and regular follow-up care.

Finally, the third category, sick patients, would be referred to a "sick-care center" consisting of clinics and hospitals, where group practice physicians would provide both intensive and acute care.

This "rational delivery system," Garfield contended, not only would save 50 percent of the time and resources of overstretched primary care physicians, it would also enable medicine to take advantage of the growing demand for medical care by keeping healthy people healthy through wellness training and basic prevention and health maintenance activities. It would result in a healthier society while maintaining an affordable system of acute care.

Garfield wasn't just fantasizing. He cited ample evidence and more was coming in from the extensive research projects then under way that pointed clearly to a new model of health care delivery. Of particular interest was a three-year study, between 1971 and 1973, that tested the effectiveness and patient acceptance of the new paramedical components of the Kaiser Permanente system, in which nurses and physician assistants were trained to carry out what today is known as "care management" programs for patients with chronic illnesses — such as diabetes, arthritis, and hypertension. The program, which emphasized health education, health maintenance and prevention, and the creation of a "continuing life record" of electronic patient information, not only led to improved outcomes, but also greatly extended the efficiency of the physicians who oversaw the paraprofessionals. Although the results were positive, the services were not yet linked with the existing primary physician care. That challenge lay on the next horizon, which became Sidney Garfield's last great research effort.

The Last Hurrah: The Total Health Care Project

Garfield named it the Total Health Care Project, best described as an effort to put into practice the delivery system he theorized about in *Scientific American*. "This project," Garfield wrote in a funding proposal, "is the next logical step." His goal was to match user demand in a large group of patients with a reorganization of traditional primary care services. Ultimately, Garfield believed that an appropriately balanced team of physicians, nurse practitioners, mental health counselors, and health educators could bring together — both effectively and economically — the entire spectrum of primary health care service.

The Total Health study, as outlined by Garfield, had a number of very specific objectives:

- Determine the well and/or sick care needs of each individual as early as possible;
- Improve access to primary care for both the well and the sick;
- Integrate into the existing primary care physician services the allied professionals required to match well and sick care needs;
- Provide each health plan member with an individualized health improvement program for optimizing health including periodic health evaluations;
- Provide management surveillance services necessary for monitoring continuity, compliance, and the health progress of each individual through time;
- Improve wellness, lifestyle behavior, and stress management;
- Conserve physician time for care of the sick;
- Provide prompt referrals to secondary care; and
- Improve member and staff satisfaction.

Finally, Garfield outlined how this new team-based approach to primary care would operate in a study with 9,270 members. The study team called in each member for a comprehensive baseline health evaluation. The results defined the personalized program needed for optimizing each individual's health. Health education advised members of things they could do to live healthier lives. A health hazard appraisal alerted each individual to his or her own unique risks — hereditary, environmental, occupational, lifestyle, or age/sex linked through time. Periodic health evaluations, scheduled according to

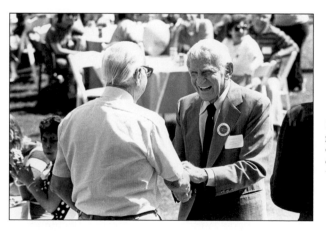

Dr. Garfield greeting a colleague at a company picnic, 1983.

need, monitored the homeostasis of physiological systems, detected early deviations, and guided health care progress over the years. Acute minor illnesses and chronic disease care follow-up was handled by protocol-guided paramedical services. The team arranged for and tracked referrals to secondary or tertiary care, maintained a central health progress data file at the team location, and continually checked on health progress and compliance with instructions and use of medications.

Work began in earnest in 1981, and by the time it was completed more than three years later, Garfield and his colleagues had tested his ideas so comprehensively that the final Total Health report filled three thick volumes.

Unfortunately, Garfield never saw those volumes. On December 29, 1984, a Saturday, he retired for the night at his home in Orinda, about 10 miles east of Oakland. He died peacefully in his sleep of an apparent heart attack.

The fact that the final report on the Total Health Care Project, the culmination of Garfield's career, was completed and published three years later is a testament to the loyalty and confidence he inspired in his colleagues, including Cecil Cutting and Morris Collen, who worked on the final report. When it was published, the dedication to Sidney Garfield read, in part:

"It was his belief that for the greatest benefit, health care should not be limited to care for the sick, but should include and emphasize the entire spectrum of prevention, health education and health maintenance ... Those of us who have had the privilege of working with him on this project find the Total Health Care study a fitting epitaph to his lifelong commitment for better health and medical care for the country."

Even so, the published study came close to following its visionary chief investigator into the grave. The report, as one observer has said, went into "hibernation." Once again, Garfield had been ahead of his time — in this case by promoting the use of paraprofessionals to perform tasks previously carried out by physicians. As Merwyn "Mitch" Greenlick, PhD, the longtime director of the Kaiser Permanente Center for Health Research in Portland, Oregon, later observed, too many Permanente doctors did not like the idea of health care teams made up of "three nurse practitioners and one physician." He said, "They wanted to have four physicians." Greenlick, who briefly worked with Garfield on some research connected with the Total Health Care Project, was among a dedicated core of Permanente leaders who saw the visionary possibilities of the work, later saying Garfield "had exactly the right model" of primary team care, "and the data out of that project proved it was cost effective."

Another physician leader, Dr. Robert Klein, the assistant physician in chief at the Oakland Medical Center during the years that the study was conducted, ultimately "rescued" the volumes of important data. In the 1990s, as Kaiser Permanente sought new ways of staying ahead of the competition by improving the primary care delivery system, Klein, by then an associate executive director of The Permanente Medical Group, led a group of 90 people in piloting new delivery models. Soon, he said, "it became clear that the voluminous data from the Total Health Care Project was more important than anything consultants could offer ..."

Already, ideas from the project had "diffused" into practice within Kaiser Permanente as a result of the experiences of physicians, nurse practitioners, and others who had worked on the research project and integrated things they had learned into practice. Klein recalled that the Total Health Care Project indeed put important ingredients for a new model "right in front of us," and he decided, "Let's really put something together where we can utilize all this knowledge that we have." Continuous work in the 1990s and in the early years of the 21st century led to an adult primary care system remarkably similar to what Garfield had envisioned — a practice that includes use of electronic medical records for each patient, primary care teams that support both patients and their personal physicians, and alternatives to the one-on-one, in-person patient visit with the doctor. These alternatives include group visits, e-mail exchanges, telephone visits, and even remote electronic monitoring. Today, the whole panoply of population-based care tools for patients with chronic conditions is essential to the adult primary care regime.

Even two decades after his death, Garfield's Total Health Care vision continued to work itself into the very definition of Kaiser Permanente. When the organization launched a major effort to reposition itself in a rapidly changing and fiercely competitive marketplace in the early years of the new century, it presented its face to the world as "a total health care organization," committed to wellness and health in all their varieties — physical, emotional, social, and even spiritual. As Klein remarked in his 2006 oral history interview, conducted by the University of California, Berkeley, "Those of us who had been around [the] Total Health Care [Project] and were at all exposed to it knew … that it worked and it was just a matter now for it to come of age. What would have happened if Sidney Garfield had never had Total Health Care I can't tell you, but I don't think we would be where we are today."

Klein's observation holds true for Garfield's entire career. Garfield did not invent preventive care or prepayment or the idea of assembling primary care physicians and specialists into multispecialty group medical practice. His genius came with his vision and his ability to assemble such innovations into a functioning *system* of care "under one roof," as he put it. That job accomplished in the first phase of his career, Garfield threw himself into hospital design, recognizing that striving for the greatest possible efficiency was one key to maintaining and improving quality, keeping medical care affordable, and expanding access to more and more people. But ultimately, Garfield came to understand that collecting, analyzing, and providing medical information at the point of care was even more important, leading him to his groundbreaking vision for computers in medicine and the Total Health Care Project. All the while, he remained sharply focused on turning sick care into health care for patients.

Were it not for Sidney Garfield, Kaiser Permanente — and the very existence of integrated health care delivery systems — would not be where it is today. Were he alive today, he would be immensely proud that Kaiser Permanente remains the nation's largest private nonprofit health care organization, with close to 9 million members cared for by more than 13,000 Permanente physicians. He would not be satisfied, however, because so much remains to be done to fulfill his vision of total health care as a right for all Americans. As he said in 1980, when asked what he would do differently if he had his life to live over, "There is nothing I would prefer doing other than what I've already done — except perhaps do a better job of it."

Toward the end of his life and after his death, Sidney Garfield was increasingly honored for his contributions to American health care. The Group Health Association of America, as early as 1969, honored him with its Distinguished Service Award. Said Dr. George Baehr, another pioneer of the group practice movement, in presenting the honor, "Not only did Dr. Garfield define the basic principles and invent the basic techniques of group practice prepayment, but he also welded them into a health care delivery system … His personal contributions to improvement of the medical face of America and indeed the world are incalculable."

In 1977, Garfield was awarded the Lyndon Baines Johnson Foundation Award, presented by Lady Bird Johnson in a ceremony in New York City. The then U.S. Secretary of Health, Education and Welfare, Joseph A. Califano, stated, "Let us hope that … we can match the sweeping vision and the earthy practicality of leaders like Sidney Garfield, who we honor today — not just for the idea he gave us, but the pioneering spirit that made that idea possible."

Not long after Garfield's death, the Henry J. Kaiser Family Foundation, which is independent of Kaiser Permanente, endowed the Sidney R. Garfield Chair in Health Sciences at the University of Southern California to honor his vision and innovation in illness prevention and health promotion. By then, Henry J. and son Edgar Kaiser were gone, too. It fell to Edgar F. Kaiser, Jr., by then chairman of the Kaiser Family Foundation, to make the presentation. Kaiser noted that, when he was born, it was Garfield who delivered him. He recalled growing up hearing debates around the dinner table about Garfield and his daring and always controversial ideas. "I usually voted for Sid," he said. "He was truly a man of vision, and those of us who did know him were blessed to know him."

❧ Appendix 1 ❧

Remarks to the AMA on Promoting Prepaid Group Practice

(Sidney Garfield, M.D., read the following slightly edited paper in a panel discussion on "Variations in Industrial Medical Service Plans" before the American Medical Association's Section on Preventive and Industrial Medicine and Public Health at the organization's annual session in Chicago, June 15, 1944. It was reprinted in the Journal of the American Medical Association, *Vol. 126, #6, pp. 337-339, Oct. 7, 1944.)*

... American medicine surpasses that of the rest of the world in technical excellence. So far a large portion of the American people has been denied this medical care. This lack of distribution has led to numerous experiments to solve the problem. During the last 10 years some 300 medical care plans have developed. This is a significant trend of vital concern to the medical profession. Most of these plans have one common characteristic — prepayment. From there on, they deviate widely in amount of coverage, financial structure, organization, and ideals.

Groups of experts have developed — so-called authorities — who are found in government agencies, foundations and labor unions, among employers, insurance companies and public health schools. Most groups are trending toward a united front, completely bypassing the medical profession — the trend toward government tax-supported medicine.

Now there appears to be a definite drive to forestall the threat of government intervention by medical society-operated prepayment plans. The facts are that prepayment itself is not enough. The majority of prepaid medical plans to date have failed and proved totally inadequate:

(a) The insurance company indemnity plans provide only a minimum of service.

(b) The Blue Cross plans have only limited hospital care and in addition have a possibility of dominating the medical profession.

(c) The medical society plans have been miserable failures. Starting with comprehensive coverage, they have dropped back to limited benefits; they have not raised the quality of medical care and are too expensive and do not provide for preventive medicine.

In short, in addition to prepayment there must be

a semblance of organization in methods of providing medical and hospital care so that the prepaid funds will provide the necessary coverage and sufficiently remunerate the physician.

Ten years ago we started providing medical care with no preconceived ideas and no plan. We had industrial work to do in areas where no medical or hospital care existed. We tried the usual method of fee-for-service and soon discarded it. We could not provide the service on that basis and the people could not pay for it. Out of our necessity evolved a simple plan that works. We have tested it under all sorts of conditions and in many areas with small numbers of men and large numbers — with scattered groups and concentrated groups. I would like to present this plan for your consideration.

The plan embodies three major principles: (1) prepayment, (2) group practice, and (3) adequate facilities. Prepayment needs no elaboration and is generally accepted as the only way people of moderate means can pay for the increasing costs of modern medical care — the principle of spreading the cost so that the well pay for the sick. Group practice, the second principle, results in many economies, the most important economy resulting from the highest quality of medical care for each illness. Most highly developed in the very universities that teach us medicine, few will deny the advantages of group practice, its stimulation to the physician, its ready accessibility for consultation, its better supervision and utilization of the younger and inexperienced physician, its productiveness in research and training. In fact, most physicians today have an unofficial association with a group of doctors; but these groups are totally unorganized, inefficient, and costly.

Adequate facilities, the third principle, are equally important. By adequate facilities I mean bringing the doctors' offices, the hospital, the laboratory and X-rays together under one roof. Where such facilities are geared to serve one particular group we achieve the utmost in efficiency and economy and the greatest accessibility among doctor, patient, and workshop, with a resulting tremendous economy in saving of travel and duplication of equipment and personnel. That, in essence, is the plan.

… You have heard and read many things about our organization. I can honestly say that the only thing wrong with what we are doing is that neither Mr. Kaiser nor I should be doing it. The doctors through their medical organizations should be doing the job. If they would, they could raise American medicine far beyond its present level, superlative as it is, and, what is more important, bring it to the people.

… Those three principles — prepayment, group practice, and adequate facilities — are the solution to medical care. There isn't a question or problem in medicine they can't answer. In effect it means organization of medical care, which has been delayed too long. It would preserve individual enterprise in medicine. Medicine has developed to the point of specialization where the individual physician can no longer be a separate enterprise. The individual group, however, can be. The free choice of the future will be the free choice of a group.

There is a tendency to be conservative and move slowly in such matters, but it would be wise in this problem to take bold steps. Group practice needs no experimentation. It has proved itself in the clinics and universities of this country. The job could be done on the basis of the state medical society and could cover all areas of the state, county and city with one statewide service. The doctors of the state could voluntarily align themselves into three groups: (1) those desiring to work in full-time group practice on a budgeted yearly income, (2) those desiring to work part time with these groups at a salary and retain some private practice, and (3) those desiring to remain in private practice ...

So all physicians could align themselves in these classes. From those volunteering for full-time group work, a board of highly trained physicians could select ideal groups or as nearly ideal as possible and back them up with part-time physicians. With careful planning, the medical centers could be built in strategic areas, city and country, serving 50 to 60 thousand people each, these centers being staffed with the groups selected. Radiating from each medical center would be the diagnostic and treatment centers, bringing readily accessible care, preventive and curative, to the outlying areas.

Such a reorganization of medicine, sponsored by the medical societies, has unlimited possibilities. Neither government, industry, nor anybody else could touch it.

Under such an arrangement medical care could easily be paid for and therefore reach all the people. There would be an increase in net income to the physicians; they would live a decent life with time off for vacations and study and home life without worrying about losing their practices. There would be a redistribution of medical care so that the country areas would be better supplied with facilities and specialties — a new hospital financial structure which would stand on its own feet and be controlled by the physicians. The younger physician coming out of training could be assured of an immediate good income and be utilized to the maximum of his capacity under supervision, and there would be a great stimulus to research and training. And very important is the fact that medical care would remain in the hands of the physician, where it belongs.

One last word: Under such an arrangement, the physician and hospital are better off if the patient never gets sick. With the modern discoveries in medicine and those yet to come, the medical care of the sick is a diminishing economy. Would it not be wiser to create now a new economy of medicine, remunerating the physician for keeping the patient well?

❧ Appendix 2 ❧

A Report on Permanente's
First 10 Years

(The following remarks are excerpted from an article by Sidney Garfield, M.D., marking the 10th anniversary of the Permanente Health Plan. It appeared in the August 1952 issue of the Permanente Foundation Medical Bulletin.)

ON HOSPITAL DESIGN

… The growth of facilities made possible achievement in another field — that of hospital and medical center designs. The Kaiser Permanente Hospitals now under construction in Los Angeles and San Francisco present many new ideas in hospital construction … By routing the public through outside corridors, an entirely new concept of hospital service is made possible. Rather than using the usual central corridor, which creates a traffic problem, the public enters the patients' rooms through sliding glass doors from the outer corridors running along outer sides of each floor. Both walls of the outside corridors are glass from floor to ceiling, affording an "outdoor" environment. Drapes operated by electric motor from the patient's bedside afford complete privacy during visiting hours.

The usual public central corridor on each floor will be restricted to physicians, nurses, and employees. It will include decentralized nurses' stations and utility rooms. Drugs, medications, X-rays, treatment materials, instruments, linens, charts, etc. for each patient will be kept at stations just outside the patient's room. Each station will be devoted to eight beds, decreasing nurses' walking to one-seventh that required under conventional floor plans. Eliminating the public from this area and decentralizing nurses' stations provides more efficient service, allows closer observation of the patient, and permits the attending physician to determine at a glance the patient's condition and treatment.

There will be a control station on each floor for a supervisor, who has direct vision of all personnel on the floor. These stations will control and route visitors down the outside corridors. The supervisor also will handle incoming and outgoing requisitions via conveyors and mail chutes, which are so planned as to serve each point for transportation of material — storeroom, pharmacy, laboratory, record room, business offices, and central supply. Requested materials are delivered automatically.

The control station will be connected with each nursing unit by intercommunication systems.

The obstetrical floor will have a built-in sound-proofed nursery behind each bed with a bassinet that is pulled through the wall separating the nursery and the mother's bed. When the bassinet is pushed back into the nursery, an automatic signal light notifies the nurse. A viewing window in the mother's room permits visitors to observe the baby in the nursery without danger to the infant. This plan caters to the principle of having the mother and baby together as much as possible for practical and psychological reasons.

The two top floors of the hospital are planned for hotel-type service for convalescent patients. As soon as patients become ambulatory, they will move to the hotel rooms where, in pleasant surroundings, they will finish out their stay. Such patients may eat in a buffet-style dining room, sleep late in the morning, participate in social recreation, watch television programs, and the like.

There will be no multiple-bed wards in the hospital. Each room will have a maximum of two beds, with many single occupancy rooms also provided. Beds will be of the electric motor type with adjustments controlled by the patient. Alongside each bed within reach of the patient will be a lavatory with hot, cold, and ice water taps, radio and phonograph outlet, piped oxygen, and individual clothes closet …

ON THE NECESSITY OF EDUCATIONAL AND RESEARCH PROGRAMS

… Permanente believed that a medical plan worthy of perpetuation, in addition to being economically sound, must provide teaching and training to stimulate high quality of care and research to contribute to medicine of the future. These objectives have been continuously stressed. Permanente has its own nursing school and its intern and approved residency training programs. A separate research laboratory building was recently acquired at Belmont, California, and a quarter of a million dollars per year has been budgeted for this program. An educational leave program has been developed for all physicians, and educational activities are encouraged. During the past year, considerable effort has been devoted to working out an affiliation with a medical school so as to develop further these educational activities.

The Permanente Foundation Hospitals offer a variety of opportunities for interns and residents to learn the art and practice of medicine. Residencies are offered in all the major specialties. The interns rotate through all the major departments. While on these services the interns take part in seminars, staff rounds and other educational conferences.

The Permanente School of Nursing was established in 1947 for the purpose of preparing young women in the art and science of nursing. Special emphasis is placed on the teaching of the methods of protecting and maintaining community health and on the skills and techniques of bedside nursing. The course of study and practice continues over a three-year period. During the first six months the student spends the greater part of her time in study. Upon completion of the preclinical period the student enters into a regimen of constant study and clinical experience in the various departments of the Permanente Hospital in Oakland, where her work is carried on under the guidance and supervision of the Oakland Hospital staff. No effort and no thought has been spared in constructing a course of studies which gives the student nurse an opportunity to acquire an excellent and basic foundation in the profession of nursing.

The research activities sponsored by Permanente fall

113

into two spheres. Clinical investigation concerned with the study of new diagnostic techniques and therapeutic agents and the development of new knowledge of disease is supported and encouraged on the part of any interested member of the medical staff. A number of research fellowships are maintained to further this work. Studies of cardiac drugs, agents for controlling the symptoms of peptic ulcer and other gastrointestinal diseases, insulin stress for the symptoms of arthritis, and medicinal agents giving promise in hypertension are examples of the projects now underway. Apart from the clinical field, Permanente pursues a program of fundamental research, which at present includes a study of the physiology of the regulation of the appetite and a project concerned with the disturbed cell chemistry in cancer and means that may possibly remedy it.

The *Permanente Foundation Medical Bulletin*, which is published periodically, is now in its 10th year. This periodical is "Dedicated to the advancement of medical care" and is composed of new contributions to the field of medical knowledge, largely from the staffs of Permanente Hospitals and the Permanente Foundation. The Educational Proceedings for the Permanente Hospitals is published 10 times a year and is essentially a record of staff lectures, educational seminars, and of proceedings at weekly grand rounds. It is intended to provide reviews and new developments in the field of medicine that may prove useful in the care of patients.

LOOKING TO THE FUTURE — OPPORTUNITY UNLIMITED

It is commonly stated that it takes 30 years to get a new idea across. Permanente's 10th anniversary marks the end of the second decade of the existence of the fundamental Permanente concept. At the start of the third decade, new horizons are opening up. The lifting of barriers to the financing of facilities, as demonstrated by the projected new construction, cannot help but make an impressive demonstration to the physicians and hospitals of the country. The excellence of these new facilities, their innovations, the quality of work being performed, the educational and research programs developed, will add in no small measure to their pyramiding evidence of worth and soundness.

We are striving to prove: (1) that high quality medical and hospital services can be rendered the people at a cost they can afford; (2) that this can be done to the benefit of all parties concerned — the people, the physicians, and the hospitals; (3) last and not least, to prove that all this can be done by private enterprise without necessity for government intervention. Any doctor can so organize his work and his companions in practice to do the same job that a Permanente medical group is doing. There is nothing sacred or secret in the idea. This cannot help but become more evident in the coming years.

There appears to be a definite acceleration evident in our progress toward these goals. The great interest displayed by doctors, labor, government, and the people in the "Permanente Idea" encourages us to believe that the accolade of "mission accomplished" cannot be too far off. It is appropriate at this time to express our appreciation to all those who have worked with us, our trustees, our physicians and fellow workers, our Health Plan members, the medical societies, civic and union leaders, and the fair opposition. Opposition to change is natural and healthy; the effect of this opposition was to stimulate us to do a better job.

⚛ Appendix 3 ⚛

From An Address to the Permanente Monterey Management Conference

(In May 1960, senior Kaiser Permanente leaders and managers met for the first interregional [Northern California, Southern California, and the Northwest] planning conference in Monterey, California to discuss strategy for the coming decade. Dr. Sidney Garfield, who had given up his leadership roles eight years earlier, seized on the occasion to urge his colleagues to move beyond the accomplishments of the past and to build "a new kind of health plan" based on computers, prevention, and wellness. The vision he first articulated in the following excerpt from that address pointed the way to the IT-enabled "total health" concept that Kaiser Permanente has pursued ever since.)

TOWARD THE TOTAL HEALTH PLAN

... I would like to use my remaining minutes on a more important, new concept. I want to throw this idea on the table for your consideration. Please accept it in the spirit it is given. It is a controversial idea, but please keep an open mind.

I think we are in a critical stage of our development. Everyone in the past few days has talked about increasing dues, labor-employer resistance, increasing

medical costs, increasing utilization, increasing old age problems, increasing capital costs — a really overwhelmingly depressing picture.

Now when you think about it, our Health Plan hasn't changed in 25 years. Except for increased dues and decreased services, it is the same old plan we dreamed about and conceived on the desert. We once called private practice horse-and-buggy medicine. I'm afraid we have a horse-and-buggy health plan ... Not only do we have a horse-and-buggy plan, but as you heard yesterday, it's not even a health plan — it's really a sick plan. All of our efforts and emphasis have been on care for the sick. It's no wonder the gap has closed, and others have imitated our plan, and we have competition. Some claim the new medical society foundation plans, such as the Stockton Plan, may be better, and we are told that Blue Cross is less costly.

It's really time for us to revitalize our plan. For the future, I suggest a radical new idea — that we stop building hospitals and clinics for sick people. Let's concentrate on a brand new type of facility — a new first in the world.

Let us conceive a building for health — designed, streamlined, and geared to serve our healthy members. This health institute could conceivably function in this fashion. Each new health plan member would automatically and periodically be called in for service. On his first visit, a history would be taken and fed in a computer. A duplicate of this history would be sent to his service area. On each periodic visit or service visit, further data would be taken from and fed into this record. This would not only develop records never before available, but might do so at a great savings in time of physicians.

Other components of this building would be a technical section where every conceivable laboratory, X-ray, EKG, and other tests could be run by such advanced new equipment as described yesterday by Mel Friedman. Again, these results would become part of the computer record.

There would be an educational section — movie rooms and lecture rooms for health education and proper use of the plan. Possibly, one would include well-baby clinics, prenatal clinics, teenage clinics, and of course, vaccinations and immunizations would be performed there. Possibly a health museum and psychiatric screening might also be included.

This idea may sound as though it might interfere with the "doctor-patient relationship" but, actually, I don't think it would. This "doctor-patient relationship" becomes important when the patient becomes sick, and the available records, the education of the member about his plan, and other features might give the physician a much sounder base for better doctor-patient relations than he has today.

It is interesting to conjecture the dream of the impact of this facility on our plan. First, it might advance us from the horse-and-buggy stage to 20 years ahead of our times again. It certainly would give our Health Plan something it has never really had — a true preventive program — something dreamed about by all plans but never accomplished before. Public relations-wise, it could sweep the country. For the first time, from the standpoint of our Health Plan representatives, they would have a definite service for the healthy member.

We have always believed that most of our turnover [lost membership] are the healthy people who haven't received much service. Now these healthy people would have received service and have a vested interest in our records and computer. We all know how wasteful and costly this turnover of membership is. This might very well reduce our turnover to nil. What this computer record of the individual, his periodic tests and symptoms could do to requirements for medical and hospital care can only be conjectured. Conceivably, it could reduce by half the need for doctors' services and hospital beds.

So, think about it. How about starting with San Jose? This might be our opportunity to reverse increasing costs and even provide care for the aged by balancing it with less expensive care for the young and healthy.

❧ Appendix 4 ❧

From An Address to the Board of Directors of The Permanente Medical Group

---

(In his address to The Permanente Medical Group Board on April 24, 1974, Dr. Sidney Garfield recounted the early history of Kaiser Permanente and then reviewed the difficult challenges and tensions of the postwar era involving his own change in status. He concluded with some inspiring advice to his fellow physicians regarding the future of the Permanente Medical Groups.)

LOOKING BACK AT A PROUD AND PAINFUL TIME

… Our health plan dropped down to almost zero [following the closing of the Kaiser Shipyards at the end of World War II], and then it began growing rather slowly. We could not advertise — information had spread by word of mouth. The [postwar public] plan grew slowly at first, gathered momentum, and after a few years, when we were sure we were going to make it, since we had built up several hundred thousand members, we felt it was time to rearrange our operations to a more permanent form following the dreams we had had at Coulee.

We set up the physicians as a separate organization and with the ideas of your partnership. We changed the health plan from my proprietorship to a nonprofit health plan, and we set up the hospital operations as nonprofit hospitals: The Permanente Medical Group, The Permanente Health Plan, and Permanente Foundation Hospitals. With that change, I divested myself of ownership and became an employee of the medical group, the health plan, and the hospitals, as the medical director of all three. I did that with complete faith — I guess you would call it blind faith — that those changes would not alter the situations that existed when I owned it. We doctors had conceived the plan, developed it, sacrificed for it, made it work, and believed that it was going to remain our operation. We felt that the nonprofit health plan and nonprofit hospitals made up a suitable framework in which we would continue to carry on our ideals. This is what everybody in our organization — all the doctors — believed, and things progressed very well during that period until around 1951, when the first Mrs. Kaiser passed away.

Mr. Kaiser soon after married one of our nurses — a very fine nurse — who actually was working as an assistant to me in my job as a medical director. With that marriage Mr. Kaiser began to show a great interest in our medical care operations. Until then he had been very busy on many other things and I could hardly get him to come through our hospital. He knew what we were doing, he helped us in any way possible, but he was rather remote from our operations.

With the marriage, this changed and he became intensely interested in our work. Out of that interest came his idea that we should build a hospital at Walnut Creek. This was a shock to all our doctors. Suddenly the organization that we doctors had built up as our own was being shaken up by others.

I went along with Mr. Kaiser on the idea of a Walnut Creek hospital. We had only 5,000 members there at that time, but it seemed like an area that would develop. I backed him up on it and even felt this would be a good way of getting him interested in this phase and possibly he would be helpful to us in the rest of our operations. But pretty soon he began to want to do things quite differently than we did them other places. He wanted Walnut Creek to be an outstanding medical center at a time when we were economizing every place else. We had started to build Southern California and San Francisco at that time, and we were being very careful and tight about the use of our funds. In addition, he wanted to select his own crew of people out there. We went along with him on that, too. Mr. and Mrs. Kaiser selected good men. But then they wanted those men to be paid different incomes than our other doctors. When we told them that wasn't possible, they decided they wanted Walnut Creek to be completely autonomous. Both of them actually believed that I had promised them that they would have an autonomous operation. What I actually did tell them was that I was blocking the things they wanted to do, and they wanted me out of the operation. I wasn't too concerned since I felt secure in my relations with the doctors, but about the same time the doctors began getting unhappy with me. They decided that I wasn't doing a good enough job as a bridge between them and Mr. Kaiser. So when both parties become unhappy and stopped backing me, I lost my job. I was kicked upstairs, put on the Board of Directors as an appeasement, I suppose, and I was given the job of planning and building facilities and taken out of operations ...

LOOKING FORWARD: LESSONS FOR THE FUTURE

... I have been asked to come up with some lessons that I have learned along the way. Those lessons may be enumerated as follows:

1) Obviously, blind faith has very definite limitations and it should be backed up with a balance of power — at least in business. Blind faith may work in religion, but it has limitations.

2) There are several kinds of power. One is the power of money, and the other is the power of solidarity of purpose. I think that I would like to pass on to you the lesson that having wealth is an extremely important point in balance of power. I have always felt strongly about this and I have always suggested that the doctors in this partnership should put away a certain number of dollars each month. I think I suggested about $200 a month. I learned the value of reserves in early years. If you had accepted that idea, you would probably have 20 or 30 million dollars by now ... Just having that wealth would give you gentlemen a great amount of power and respect in

dealing with other people. It is one of the things that matters in this world.

The other power you should have is the power of acting together, the power of what I call solidarity. You can fight among yourselves, but as far as the outside world is concerned, have one common face and purpose just as you would in your own family. I think that if you would have a federation with the doctors in Southern California and the other regions, if possible, you would have all the power you need to control your destiny in the future. I don't think anything will ever happen again, but it would do you no harm and it would be wise to build up your strength — through federation, or wealth, or both.

3) Most important of all, I think you ought to build up your competitive position in this medical world by innovation and opening up to change. We have been doing the same thing far too long. Some of you have heard that talk I gave on the new Medical Care Delivery System. That may not be the only answer, but it is a move to improve service. You should be getting into that — improving service. You know institutions tend to become static; they build walls around themselves to protect themselves from change, and eventually die. You should fight that by opening up your thinking and your ideas, and work for a change. Improvement of service is very important for the competition you face in the future. I think you should try to divert construction money and renovation money; put them off for awhile; put your money into more and better service to the people. That is where it is needed ... I would urge you to get on with it as soon as possible.

So in plain words I give you this advice. Keep your feet on the ground, keep your hands on your purses, make sure your operations are as economical as possible, and build up your wealth for strength. Keep your arms on each other's shoulders and keep your eyes on the stars for innovation and change for the future. I am not sure that that last point, improvement of service, won't be your greatest strength if you really work at it.

❧ Appendix 5 ❧

The Delivery of Medical Care

Medical care in the U.S. is expensive and poorly distributed, and national health insurance will make things worse. What is needed is an innovative system in which the sick are separated from the well.

By Sidney R. Garfield, M.D.

The U.S. system of high-quality but expensive and poorly distributed medical care is in trouble. Dramatic advances in medical knowledge and new techniques, combined with soaring demands created by growing public awareness, by hospital and medical insurance and by Medicare and Medicaid, are swamping the system by which medical care is delivered. As the disparity between the capabilities of medical care and its availability increases, and as costs rise beyond the ability of most Americans to pay them, pressures build up for action. High on the list of suggested remedies are national health insurance and a new medical care delivery system.

National health insurance, an attractive idea to many Americans, can only make things worse. Medicare and Medicaid — equivalents of national health insurance for segments of our population — have largely failed because the surge of demand they created only dramatized and exacerbated the inadequacies of the existing delivery system and its painful shortages of manpower and facilities. It is folly to believe that compounding this demand by extending health insurance to the entire population will improve matters. On the contrary, it is certain that further overtaxing of our inadequate medical resources will result in serious deterioration in the quality and availability of service for the sick. If this country has learned anything from experience with Medicare and Medicaid, it is that a rational delivery system should have been prepared for projects of such scope.

The question then becomes: What are the necessary elements of a rational medical care delivery system? Many have proposed that prepaid group practice patterned after the Kaiser Permanente program, a private system centered on the West Coast, may be a solution. We at Kaiser Permanente, who have had more than 30 years' experience working with health care problems, believe that prepaid group practice is a step in the right direction but that it is far from being the entire answer. Lessons we have learned lead us to believe there is a broader solution that is applicable both to the Kaiser Permanente system and to the system of private practice that prevails today.

The heart of the traditional medical care delivery system is the physician. Whether he practices alone or in a group, he is still directly involved in the care of the patient at every important stage, from the initial interview to the final discharge. Any realistic solution to the medical care problem must therefore begin by facing up to the facts about the supply of physicians.

Of the active doctors in the U.S. a great many are engaged in research, teaching, and administration. Those actually giving patient care, in practice and on hospital staffs, number about 275,000 (approximately 135 per 100,000 of population), and they are far from evenly distributed throughout the population. A preponderance are in urban areas, and within those areas they tend to be concentrated where people can best afford their services. Increasing specialization accentuates the shortage of doctors. If we were to augment the output of our medical schools from the present level (fewer than 9,000 doc-tors a year) to twice that number (which is scarcely possible), we would barely affect this supply in 20 years, considering the natural attrition in our existing physician complement. The necessity of living with a limited supply of physicians in the face of increasing demand forces us to focus on the need for a medical care delivery system that utilizes scarce and costly medical manpower properly.

The traditional medical care delivery system has evolved over the years with little deliberate planning. At the end of the 19th century medical care was still relatively primitive: there was the doctor and his black bag and there were hospitals — place to die. People generally stayed away from the doctor unless they were very ill. In this century expanding medical knowledge soon became too much for any one man to master, and specialties began developing. Laboratories, X-ray facilities, and hospitals became important adjuncts to the individual physician in his care of sick people. Since World War II a chain reaction of accelerated research, expanding knowledge, important discoveries, and new technology has brought medical care to the level of a sophisticated discipline, offering much hope in the treatment of illness, yet requiring the precise and costly teamwork of specialists operating in expensively equipped and highly organized facilities (see Figures 1a and 1b).

Throughout these years of remarkable medical achievement the delivery system has remained relatively unchanged, as though oblivious to the great need for new forms of organization equal to the task of applying new techniques and knowledge. Physicians have clung to individualism and old traditions. Their individual hospitals have continued on their individual ways, striving to be all things to their doctors and patients, creating their own private domains, largely ignoring the tremendous need to merge their highly specialized services and facilities. It is only in comparatively recent years that group practice by doctors has been considered respectable (and as yet only some 12 percent of all physicians practice in groups) and that regional facility planning boards have appeared

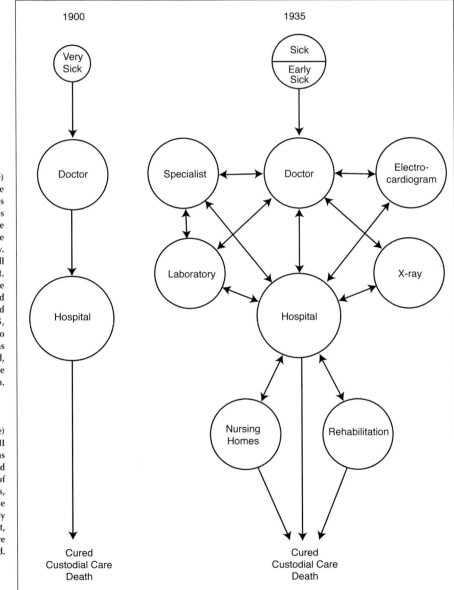

Figure 1a. (this page) Medical care has become more complex in this century, and as it has become more effective the entry mix of people has changed significantly. Yet the entry point is still the doctor's appointment. Before 1900 medicine had little to offer and only sick people entered medical care. By 1935, as medicine began to have more to offer and as insurance plans appeared, some "early sick" people were entering the system.

Figure 1b. (next page) Since World War II medical technology has proliferated, as indicated by the partial display of treatment components, and more well people enter the mix largely because of prepayment, insurance plans, Medicare and Medicaid.

to force some semblance of cooperation on hospital construction.

It is amazing that the traditional delivery system functioned as well as it did for so long, considering the stresses between old methods and new technology. Much of its inefficiency was absorbed by dedicated physicians working long hours and donating additional hours; much was absorbed by office and

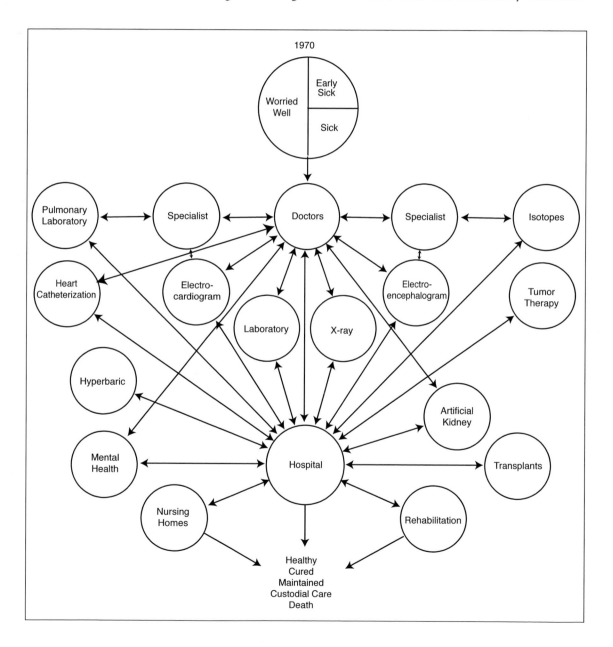

hospital personnel working for extremely low pay. Only recently, under the joint impact of soaring demands for service and demands for competitive wages, has the system begun to break down, but it has been faltering for some time. In 1967, the National Advisory Commission on Health Manpower reported that "medical care in the U.S. is more a collection of bits and pieces (with overlapping, duplication, great gaps, high costs and wasted effort) than an integrated system in which need and efforts are closely related."

Let us look at another medical care delivery system: the Kaiser Permanente plan. This program had its origin in southern California in the depression years from 1933 to 1938. I was then in private practice, and I became involved in providing medical and hospital services and facilities for several thousand construction workers. Unable to make ends meet by depending for remuneration on the usual fee for service, I finally tried prepayment and thus happened on our basic concepts of health care. Prepayment to a group of physicians in integrated clinic and hospital facilities proved to be a remarkably effective system for providing comprehensive care to workers on a completely self-sustaining basis. At the Grand Coulee Dam from 1938 to 1942, with the warm interest and counsel of Henry J. Kaiser and his son Edgar, these basic concepts were further developed, tested, and broadened into a complete family plan for the entire temporary community built around that construction job.

World War II expanded our Health Plan concept into care for 90,000 workers of the Kaiser wartime shipyards in the San Francisco Bay area and a similar number of workers in the Portland and Vancouver area. At the end of the war these workers returned to their homes, leaving us with facilities and medical and hospital organizations. We decided to make our services available to the community at large. Since 1945 the plan has grown of its own impetus, without advertising, to its present size: more than two million subscribers served by outpatient centers, 51 clinics and 22 hospitals in California, Oregon, Washington, and Hawaii and in Cleveland and Denver. The plan provides comprehensive care at an annual cost of $100 per capita, which is approximately two-thirds the cost of comparable care in most parts of the country.

The plan is completely self-sustaining. Physical facilities and equipment worth $267 million have been financed by Health Plan income and bank loans (except for gifts and loans to the extent of about 2 percent). The plan income provides funds for teaching, training, and research, and pays competitive incomes to 2,000 physicians and 13,000 non-physician employees.

The Health Plan and the hospitals are organized as nonprofit operations and the medical groups in each area are autonomous partnerships. This organization gives our physicians essentially the same incentives as physicians in private practice have; they are motivated, in addition, by their belief in the rightness of this way of practicing medicine.

In addition to prepayment, group practice, and the integration of hospital and clinic facilities, we can identify three other principles that are essential to the plan's success. One is the institution of what is in effect a new medical economics, which flows simply from the fact that the total Health Plan income is turned over to the physicians and hospitals not as a fee for specific services but as a total sum. This reverses the usual economics of medicine: our doctors are better off if our subscribers stay well and our hospitals better off if their beds are empty. Another principle is freedom of choice. We require any group that wants to enroll its members in our group to offer them at least one alternative choice of medical plan, be it Blue Cross or a medical society plan, or something else. Finally, we consider it a fundamental principle that the physicians must be involved in responsibility for administrative and operational decisions that affect the quality of the care they provide.

We believe any group of physicians, or a foundation working with physicians, can easily duplicate the Kaiser Permanente success. It only requires a dedicated group of physicians with reasonably well-organized facilities, a membership desiring their services on a prepaid basis, and strict adherence to all these principles.

All of this is not to say that U.S. medicine should change over to the Kaiser Permanente pattern. On the contrary, freedom of choice is important; we believe that the choice of alternate systems, including solo practice, is preferable for both the public and physicians. Any change to prepaid group practice should be evolutionary, not revolutionary. Physicians in general have too much time and effort vested in their practice to discard them overnight. It will probably be the younger men, starting out in practice, who will innovate. Medical school faculties should point out the advantages and disadvantages of all methods of practice to these young men so that they can choose wisely.

Let us examine the functioning of these two systems — the traditional system and the Kaiser Permanente one. In the language of systems analysis, the traditional medical care system has an input (the patient), a processing unit of discrete medical resources (individual doctors and individual hospitals) and an output (one hopes the cured or improved patient). Customarily the patient decides when he needs care. This more or less educated decision by the patient creates a variable entry mix into medical care consisting of 1) the well, 2) the "worried well," 3) the "early sick," and 4) the sick. This entry mix has markedly increased in quantity and changed in character over the years as medical care resources have grown in complexity and specialization. One constant throughout this evolution has been the point of entry into the system, which is and always has been the appointment with the doctor. Moreover, in traditional practice the patient enters with a fee.

The Kaiser Permanente program alters the traditional medical care delivery system in only two ways. It eliminates the fee for service, substituting prepayment, and it organizes the many units of medical care resources into a coordinated group practice in integrated clinic and hospital facilities. We have come to realize that ironically the elimination of the fee has created a new set of problems. The lessons we have learned in seeking to solve these problems have a direct bearing on the difficulties besetting the country's faltering medical care system.

The obvious purpose of the fee is remuneration of the physician. It has a less obvious but very significant side effect: it is a potent regulator of flow into the delivery system. Since nobody wants to pay for unneeded medical care, one tends to put off seeing the doctor until one is really sick. This limits the number of people seeking entry, particularly the number of well and early-sick people. Conversely, the sicker a person is, the earlier he seeks help — regardless of fee. Thus, the fee-for-service regulator tends to limit overall quantity, to decrease the number of the healthy and early sick and to increase the number of the really sick in the entry mix.

Elimination of the fee has always been a must in our thinking, since it is a barrier to early entry into sick care. Early entry is essential for early treatment and for preventing serious illness and complications. Only after years of costly experience did we discover that the elimination of the fee is practically as much of a barrier to early sick care as the fee itself. The reason is that when we removed the fee, we removed the regulator of flow into the system and put nothing in its place. The result is an uncontrolled flood of well, worried-well, early-sick, and sick people into our point of entry — the doctor's appointment — on a first-come, first-served basis that has little relation to priority of need. The impact of this demand overloads the system and, since the well and worried-well people are a considerable proportion of our entry mix, the usurping of available doctors' time by healthy people actually interferes with the care of the sick.

The same thing has happened at the broad national level. The traditional medical care delivery system, which has evolved rather loosely over the years subject to the checks and balances of the open market, is being overwhelmed because of the elimination of personally paid fees through the spread of health insurance, Medicare, and Medicaid. This floods the system not only with increased numbers of people but also with a changed entry mix characterized by an increasing proportion of relatively well people. For this considerable segment of patients the old methods of examining and diagnosing used by the doctor become very inefficient. He spends a large portion of his time trying to find something wrong with healthy people by applying the techniques he was taught for diagnosing illness. This reverse use of sick-care technology for healthy and comparatively symptomless people is wasteful of the doctor's time and boring and frustrating for him.

The obvious solution is to find a new regulator to replace the eliminated fee at the point of entry, one that is more sensitive to real medical need than to ability to pay and that can help to separate the well from the sick and establish entry priorities for the sick. We believe we have developed just such a regulator. Our Medical Methods Research Department, headed by Morris F Collen, who is an electrical engineer as well as a physician, has successfully developed and tested techniques for evaluating the health of our members. The system that has been developed, which is variously called multiphasic screening, health evaluation, or simply health testing, promises to solve the problem of a new regulator to flow into our medical care delivery system.

Originally designed to meet our ever-increasing demand for periodic health checkups, health testing combines a detailed computerized medical history with a comprehensive panel of physiological tests administered by paramedical personnel. Tests record the function of the heart, thyroid, neuromuscular system, respiratory system, vision, and hearing. Other tests record height and weight, blood pressure, a urine analysis, and a series of 20 blood-chemistry measurements plus hematology. The chest and (in women) the breasts are X-ray'd. By the time the entire process is completed the computerized results generate "advice" rules that recommend further tests when needed or, depending on the urgency of any significant abnormalities, an immediate or routine appointment with a physician. The entire record is stored by the computer as a health profile for future reference.

This health-testing procedure is ideally suited to be a regulator of entry into medical care. Certainly it is more sophisticated than the usual fee for service or our present first-come, first-served method. As a new entry regulator, health testing serves to separate the well from the sick and to establish entry priorities. In addition it detects symptomless and early illness, provides a preliminary survey for the doctors, aids in the diagnostic process, provides a basic health profile for future reference, saves the doctor (and patient) time and visits, saves hospital days for diagnostic work, and makes possible the maximum utilization of paramedical personnel. Most important of all, it falls into place as the heart of a new and rational medical care delivery system (see Figure 2).

As I have indicated, much of the trouble with the existing delivery system derives from the impact of an unstructured entry mix on scarce and valuable doctor time. Health testing can effectively sepa-

rate this entry mix into its basic components: the healthy, the symptomless early sick, and the sick. This clear separation is the key to the rational allocation of needed medical resources to each group. With health testing as the heart of the system, the entry mix is sorted into its components, which fan out to each of three distinct divisions of service: a health care service, a preventive maintenance service, and a sick care service. Compare this with the existing process, where the entire heterogeneous entry mix empties into the doctor's appointment, a sick care service.

Health care service is a new division of medicine that does not exist in this country or in any other country. Medical planners have long dreamed of the day when resources and funds could be channeled into keeping people healthy, in contrast to our present overwhelming preoccupation with curing sickness. Yet health care has been an elusive concept, and understandably so: well people entering medical care have been hopelessly mixed into and submerged in sick care, the primary concern of doctors. Doctors trained and oriented to sick care have been much too busy to be involved in the care of well people. True health care never had a chance to develop in that environment. In fact, not even the highly socialized governments with socialized medicine have created any significant services for the healthy other than sanitation and immunization. These governments swamp the doctor with the entire entry mix of well and sick and thus are unable to provide adequate care for either.

The clear definition of a health care service, made possible by health testing, is a basic first step toward a positive program for keeping people well. It should be housed in a new type of health facility where in pleasant surroundings lectures, health exhibits, audio-visual tapes and films, counseling, and other services would be available. Whether or not one believes in the possibility of actually keeping people well, however, is now beside the point; this new health care service is absolutely

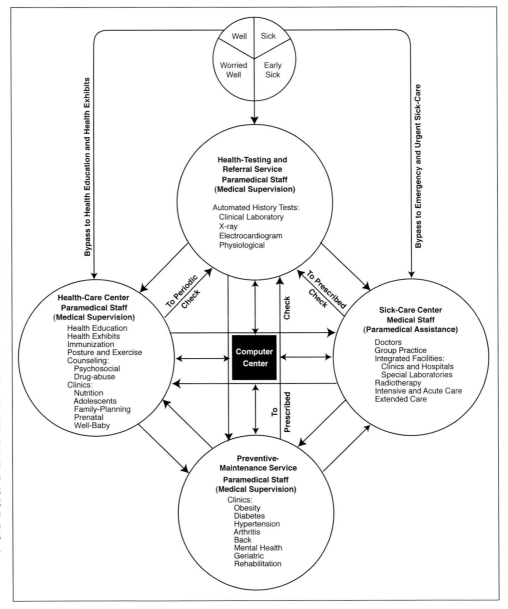

Figure 2. New delivery system proposed by the author would separate the sick from the well. It would do this by establishing a new method of entry, the health-testing service, to perform the regulating function that was performed, more crudely, by the fee for service. After health testing the patient would be referred for sick care, health care, or preventive maintenance as required and would be transferred among the services as his condition changed. The computer center would regulate the flow of patients and information among the units, coordinating the entire system, which would depend heavily on paramedical personnel to save doctors' time.

essential in order to meet the increasing demand for just this kind of service and to keep people from overloading sick care resources.

Preventive maintenance service, like health care service, has been submerged in sick care. Essentially it is a service for high-incidence chronic illness that requires routine treatment, monitoring, and follow-up; its object is to improve the patient's condition or prevent progression of the illness, if possible, and to guard against complications. This type of care, performed by paramedical personnel reporting to the patient's doctor, can save a great deal of the doctor's time and (because it allows more frequent visits) provide closer and better surveillance.

The use of paramedical personnel with limited knowledge and limited but precise skills to relieve the physician of minor routine and repetitious tasks requires that such tasks be clearly defined and well supervised. Procedures are automatically defined and structured in the new system by the clear separation of services. Three of the four divisions of the proposed system — health testing services, health care services and preventive maintenance service — are primarily areas of paramedical personnel. Supervising physicians will be involved in varying degrees: least in health testing and most in preventive maintenance. This leaves sick care, with its judgments on diagnosis and treatment, clearly in the physician's realm. Even here, however, he will be aided by the three other services: in diagnosis, by health testing; in follow-up care, by preventive maintenance; in repetitive explanations and instructions to patients and relatives, by the audiovisual library of the health

care service. We believe, incidentally, that the doctor-patient relationship, which is suffering from the pressure of crowded schedules today, would gain under this system. Giving the doctor more time for care of the sick can help to preserve the relationship at the stage where it counts most.

Implementing the new delivery system should be relatively simple in the Kaiser Permanente program, since there are no basic conflicts: The subscribers will benefit from better and prompter service to both the well and the sick; the doctors will have more time for their sick patients and their work will be more interesting and stimulating. Although the complete system remains to be tested and evaluated at each step, our hypothesis, on the basis of our research to date, is that we can save at least 50 percent of our general practitioners', internists' and pediatricians' time. This should greatly enhance our service for the sick and improve our services for the well.

Implementing this new medical care delivery system in the world of traditional medical practice will be more difficult, but it still makes sense. Many forward-looking physicians will see in these new methods an opportunity to improve their services to patients. Most doctors these days have more work than they can handle and begrudge the time they must spend on well people. The assistance they could get from health testing and health care services will be welcome to many of them if such services are carefully designed and planned to help them. The sponsorship of health testing and health care services for private practice logically falls to the local medical societies. Some have already moved in the direction of health evaluation. A few local medical societies in northern California have for several years been operating a mobile unit evaluating the health of cannery workers. Some leaders of other medical societies have expressed interest in health testing as an entry into medical care. They realize that improvement of the delivery system is essential for the preservation of the private enterprise of medicine in this country.

The proposed delivery system may offer a solution to the hitherto insoluble problem of poverty medical care in many areas. The need is to make health services accessible to poor people. To this end neighborhood clinics are established, but staffing these clinics with physicians has proved virtually impossible. Physicians in general want to be in a stimulating medical environment; they like to associate with well-trained colleagues in good medical centers and tend to avoid isolated clinics.

In the system being proposed a central medical center, well staffed and equipped, would provide sick care. It could have four or five "outreach" neighborhood clinics, each providing the three primarily paramedical services: health testing, health care, and preventive maintenance. Staffing these services with paramedical personnel should be much less difficult than staffing clinics with doctors; many of the workers could be recruited from the neighborhood itself. Such outreach clinics, coordinated with the sick-care center, could provide high-quality, personal service — better service, perhaps, than is available to the affluent today — at a cost probably lower than the cost of the inferior service poor people now receive.

The concept of medical care as a right is an excellent principle that both the public and the medical world have now accepted. Yet the words mean very little, since we have no system capable of delivering quality medical care as a right. This is hardly surprising. Picture what would happen to, say, transportation service if fares were suddenly eliminated and travel became a right. What would happen to our already overtaxed airports and what chance would anyone have of getting anywhere if he really needed to? National health insurance, if it were legislated today, would have the same effect. It would create turmoil. Even if sick care were superbly organized today, with group practice in well-integrated facilities, the change from "fee" to "free" would stagger the system.

Quality medical care as a right cannot be achieved unless we can establish need, separate the well from the sick, and do that without wasting physicians' time. It follows that to make medical care a right, or national health insurance possible, it is mandatory that we first make available health testing and health care services throughout the country. It is our conviction that these services should be provided or arranged for by the physicians themselves in order to be responsive to their needs and not just a commercial operation.

A basic cause-and-effect relationship is directly responsible for much of today's medical care problems. The cause is the elimination of a personally paid fee for medical service. The effect is a changed, unstructured entry mix into the delivery system that wastes scarce medical manpower. The suggested solution, a new method of entry through health testing, serves as the heart of a new medical care delivery system for the future.

The entry of healthy people into the medical care system should not be considered undesirable. It opens the door to a great opportunity for American medicine: If these well people are guided away from sick care into a new, meaningful health care service, there is hope that we can develop an effective preventive-care program for the future. The concomitant release of misused doctors' time can significantly slow the trend toward the inflation of costs and mal-distribution and unavailability of service. There should be little shortage of manpower if manpower is utilized properly.

Medical care stands at a critical point. One choice would be to adopt rash legislation that can only depreciate the quality of care for both the sick and the well. The better choice is to create a rational new medical care delivery system that will make it genuinely possible to achieve the principle of quality medical care as a right. Matching the superb technology of present-day medicine with an effective delivery system can raise U.S. medical care to a level unparalleled in the world.

⚘ Bibliography ⚘

Allen, Terri Ann. *SCPMG ... The First Fifty Years: History of the Southern California Permanente Medical Group, 1953-2003.* Los Angeles: Southern California Permanente Medical Group, 2003.

Barton, Jane. "Good Nursing Is Core of Panorama Plan." *The Modern Hospital* 99 November 1962: 86-91.

Bolotin, Sally. Interview by Steve Gilford, Sherman Oaks, CA, August 29, 2006.

Breslow, Lester. *A Life in Public Health: An Insider's Retrospective.* New York: Springer Publishing Co., 2004.

Cadman, Paul F. Manuscript. "The Builder: The Life and Work of Henry J. Kaiser." Kaiser Permanente Heritage Resources Archive, Oakland, CA.

Champion, Hale. "Health Plan Controversy: How the New Kaiser Hospital Works." *San Francisco Chronicle*, February 14-16, 1954.

———. "Henry J. Kaiser: New Kind of Medicine Man." *The Progressive* June 1954: 21ff.

Collen, Morris F., ed. *Multiphasic Health Testing Services.* New York: John Wiley & Sons, 1978.

———. "History of the Kaiser Permanente Medical Care Program," an Oral History Interview Conducted in 1986 by Sally Smith Hughes. Berkeley, CA: Regional Oral History Office, The Bancroft Library, University of California, Berkeley, 1988.

Cutting, Cecil C. "History of the Kaiser Permanente Medical Care Program," an Oral History Interview Conducted in 1985 by Malca Chall. Berkeley, CA: Regional Oral History Office, The Bancroft Library, University of California, Berkeley, 1986.

Cutting, Cecil C., and Morris F. Collen. "A Historical Review of the Kaiser Permanente Medical Care Program." *Journal of the Society for Health Systems*, 3, no. 4 (1992): 25-30.

Daniels, Mark. "The Permanente Foundation Hospital." *Architect and Engineer* May 1945, 10ff.

Davies, Lawrence E. *A World War II Diary.* Hat Creek, CA: HiStory Ink Books, 1994.

Debley, Tom. "KP HealthConnect: Fulfilling the Vision of KP's Founding Physician." *The Permanente Journal* 8, no. 4 (2004):32-3.

———. "Think the Unthinkable, Dream the Impossible." An address delivered at The History of Medicine Society at The Oregon Health & Science University, Portland, OR, January 2006.

de Kruif, Paul. *Kaiser Wakes the Doctors.* New York: Harcourt Brace, 1943.

———. "Tomorrow's Health Plan—Today!" *Reader's Digest*, May 1943, 61ff.

———. "Many Will Rise and Walk." *Reader's Digest*, February 1946, 79 ff.

———. *Life Among the Doctors.* New York: Harcourt Brace, 1949.

Dusheck, George. "Henry Kaiser's Big Medicine Is Now Fifteen Years Old." *San Francisco News*, October 29, 1957.

Engel, Jonathan. *Doctors and Reformers: Discussion and Debate Over Health Policy, 1925-1950.* Columbia, SC: University of South Carolina Press, 2002.

Fleming, Scott. "Evolution of the Kaiser-Permanente Medical Care Program: An Historical Overview." Kaiser Permanente Heritage Resources Archive, Oakland, CA, 1982.

———. "History of the Kaiser Permanente Medical Care Program," an Oral History Interview Conducted in 1990 and 1991 by Sally Smith Hughes. Berkeley, CA: Regional Oral History Office, The Bancroft Library, University of California, Berkeley, 1997.

Foster, Mark S. *Henry J. Kaiser: Builder of the Modern American West.* Austin: University of Texas Press, TX, 1989.

Fowler, Dan. "More Care for Less Money: Henry J. Kaiser's Medical Plan." *Look*, Sept. 9, 1952, 73-5.

———. "Push-Button Hospital." *Look*, December 15, 1953, 92 *passim.*

Gilliam, Harold. "A Revolutionary Medical Plan Comes to the Waterfront." *San Francisco Chronicle*, July 15, 1951.

Han, Paul K. J. "Historical Changes in the Objectives of the Periodic Health Examination." *Annals of Internal Medicine*, 127, no. 10 (November 1997): 910-7.

Heiner, Albert P. *Henry J. Kaiser: Western Colossus*. San Francisco: Halo Books, 1991.

Hendricks, Rickey. "Medical Practice Embattled: Kaiser Permanente, the American Medical Association, and Henry J. Kaiser on the West Coast, 1945-1955." *The Pacific Historical Review*, 60, no. 4 (November 1991): 439-73.

———. *A Model for National Health Care: The History of Kaiser Permanente*. New Brunswick, NJ: Rutgers University Press, 1993.

Kaiser, Henry J. Address to Physicians at the St. Francis Hotel, San Francisco, CA, June 9, 1948.

———. "The New Economics of Medical Care." An address to the National Press Club, Washington, D.C., May 26, 1954.

Kay, Raymond M. *Historical Review of Southern California Permanente Medical Group: Its Role in the Development of the Kaiser Permanente Medical Care Program in Southern California*. Los Angeles: Southern California Permanente Medical Group, 1979.

———. "History of the Kaiser Permanente Medical Care Program," an Oral History Interview Conducted in 1985 by Ora Huth. Berkeley, CA: Regional Oral History Office, The Bancroft Library, University of California, Berkeley, 1987.

Keene, Clifford H. "History of the Kaiser Permanente Medical Care Program," an Oral History Interview Conducted in 1985 by Sally Smith Hughes. Berkeley, CA: Regional Oral History Office, The Bancroft Library, University of California, Berkeley, 1986.

Kuh, Clifford. "The Permanente Health Plan for Industrial Workers." *Industrial Medicine* 14, no. 4 (April 1945): 3 ff.

Lane, Frederick C. *Ships for Victory: A History of Shipbuilding Under the U.S. Maritime Commission in World War II by Frederick C. Lane with the Collaboration of Blanche D. Coll, Gerald J. Fischer, David B. Tyler, and Joseph T. Reynolds*. Baltimore: Johns Hopkins University Press, 2001.

Lindbergh, Alma. Manuscript. "History of the Kaiser Organizations." Kaiser Permanente Heritage Resources Archive, Oakland, CA.

Martin, Helen Eastman. *The History of the Los Angeles County Hospital (1878-1968) and the Los Angeles County-University of Southern California Medical Center (1968-1978)*. Los Angeles: University of Southern California Press, 1979.

Ordway, Alonzo B. Interview by Dan Scannell, Oakland, CA, 1967.

Saward, Ernest, W. "History of the Kaiser Permanente Medical Care Program," an Oral History Interview Conducted in 1985 by Sally Smith Hughes. Berkeley, CA: Regional Oral History Office, The Bancroft Library, University of California, Berkeley, 1986.

———. "Lessons and Parables in Health Care: A Tale of Two Cities." The First Annual Ernest W. Saward Lecture. Portland, OR: Kaiser Permanente Center for Health Research, 1989.

Shelby, Betty. "The Modern Hospital of the Month [Kaiser Foundation Medical Center, Honolulu, HI]: Central Work Corridor Simplifies Nurses' Work." *The Modern Hospital* 93 (December 1959): 65-70.

Smillie, John G. "History of the Kaiser Permanente Medical Care Program," an Oral History Interview Conducted in 1985 by Ora Huth. Berkeley, CA: Regional Oral History Office, The Bancroft Library, University of California, Berkeley, 1987.

———. *Can Physicians Manage the Quality and Costs of Health Care? The Story of the Permanente Medical Group*. New York: McGraw-Hill, 1991.

Somers, Anne R., ed. *Kaiser-Permanente Medical Care Program: One Valid Solution to the Problem of Health Care Delivery in the U.S. A Symposium*. New York: The Commonwealth Fund, 1971.

Starr, Kevin. *Embattled Dreams: California in War and Peace, 1940-1950*. Oxford: Oxford University Press, 2002.

Starr, Paul. *The Social Transformation of American Medicine*. New York: Basic Books, 1982.

U.S. House Committee on Interstate and Foreign Commerce. Henry J. Kaiser. "A Private Enterprise Solution to Medical Care by the Doctors of this Country." 83rd Cong., 2nd Sess., January 11, 1954.

Velie, Lester. "Supermarket Medicine." *The Saturday Evening Post*, June 20, 1953, 22 *passim*.

War Manpower Commission. *Physical Demands and Capacities Analysis*. San Francisco and Oakland: War Manpower Commission and Permanente Foundation Hospitals, 1944.

Weeks, Lewis E. ed. *Ernest W. Saward, In First Person: An Oral History*. Hospital Administration Oral History Collection. Chicago: American Hospital Association, 1987.

Williams, Greer. "Kaiser." *Modern Hospital* 116 (February 1971): 67-95.

Wolf, Donald E. *Big Dams and Other Dreams: The Six Companies Story*. Norman, OK: University of Oklahoma Press, 1996.

Yedidia, Avram. "History of the Kaiser Permanente Medical Care Program," an Oral History Interview Conducted in 1985 by Ora Huth. Berkeley, CA: Regional Oral History Office, The Bancroft Library, University of California, Berkeley, 1987.

Zoloth, Laurie. "The Best Laid Plans: Resistant Community and the Intrepid Vision in the History of Managed Care Medicine." *Journal of Medicine and Philosophy*, 24, no. 5 (1999): 461-491.

❧ Selected Works ❧

Authored or Coauthored
by Sidney R. Garfield, M.D.

Collected together for the first time, the *Sidney R. Garfield, M.D. Papers* at the Kaiser Permanente Heritage Resources Archive support research into Garfield's role as co-founder of Kaiser Permanente and his contributions to the theory and practice of health care delivery systems. These papers are available for review at the Heritage Resources Archive by appointment.

Collen, F. Bobbie, Robert Feldman, Krikor Soghikian, and Sidney R. Garfield. "The Educational Adjunct to Multiphasic Health Testing." *Preventive Medicine* 2, no. 2 (June 1973): 247-60.

Collen, Francis Bobbie, Blanche Madero, Krikor Soghikian, and Sidney R. Garfield. "Kaiser Permanente Experiment in Ambulatory Care." *American Journal of Nursing* 71, no. 7 (July 1971): 1371-4.

Collen, Morris F., Sidney R. Garfield, and James H. Duncan. "The Multiphasic Checkup for Evaluation of Well People." In *Challenges and Prospects for Advanced Medical Systems*. Miami: Symposia Specialists, 1978.

Collen, Morris F., S. R. Garfield, Robert H. Richart, James H. Duncan, and Robert Feldman. "Cost Analyses of Alternative Health Examination Modes." *Archives of Internal Medicine* 137, no. 1 (January 1977): 73-9.

Feldman, R., S. L. Taller, Sidney R. Garfield, and others. "Nurse Practitioner Multiphasic Health Checkups." *Preventive Medicine* 6 (1977): 391-403.

Garfield, Sidney R. *Papers*. Kaiser Permanente Heritage Resources Archive, Oakland, CA.

———. "The Essential Features Of The Kaiser Plan." *Journal of the American Medical Association* 125 (1944): 188.

———. "Health Plan Principles in the Kaiser Industries." *Journal of the American Medical Association* 126, no. 6 (1944): 337-9.

———. "First Annual Report of Permanente Foundation Hospital." *Permanente Foundation Medical Bulletin*, II, no. 1 (January 1944): 35-48.

———. "Address to the Multnomah County Medical Association." Portland, OR, April 4, 1945.

———. "Group Medicine: A Discussion of the Economics of Medical Care—It Works at Permanente." *Modern Hospital* 45 (November 1945): 53-5.

———. "The Plan That Kaiser Built." *Survey Graphic*, December 1945, 480-2.

———. "A Report on Permanente's First Ten Years." *Permanente Foundation Medical Bulletin* X, nos. 1-4 (August 1952): 1-11.

———. *Statement of Sidney R. Garfield Concerning Protection Against Catastrophic Diseases*. U.S. House Committee on Interstate and Foreign Commerce. Sidney R. Garfield. Washington, DC. 83rd Cong., 2nd Sess., January 6, 1954.

———. "The Kaiser Foundation Health Plan." *The Prescriber*, November 1954.

———. "Kaiser Foundation Health Plan." Remarks before the California State Assembly Interim Committee on Finance and Insurance, San Francisco, November 3-4, 1955.

———. "Address by Sidney R. Garfield, M.D., Kaiser Foundation Hospitals of Northern California Fifteenth Anniversary."

Commemorative address on the occasion of the fifteenth anniversary of Kaiser Foundation Hospitals of Northern California, Berkeley, CA, October 19, 1957.

———. Address to the Kaiser Foundation Hospitals Panel, the Monterey Management Conference, Monterey, CA, May 11, 1960.

———. Address to the Pack Forest Conference, the University of Washington, Seattle, WA, October 3, 1964.

———. "Medicine of the Future." Address to the Staff Education Conference for Physicians, San Mateo, CA, October 31, 1965.

———. "Rationally Organized Medicine." Draft, audience unknown, November 16, 1966.

———. Address to the Medical Entities Management Association, Kaiser Foundation Hospitals of Southern California, February 1969.

———. "Where Goes the Kaiser Foundation Health Plan?" Address to the Permanente Physician Orientation Communications Session, Oakland, CA, October 3-4, 1969.

———. Address to the Group Health Association of America Annual Luncheon, American Public Health Association, Philadelphia, PA, November 12, 1969.

———. "The Delivery of Medical Care." *Scientific American* 222, no. 4 (April 1970): 15ff.

———. "Kaiser Permanente's Prepaid Plan." Address to the Utah State Medical Association, Salt Lake City, UT, September 9, 1970.

———. "What We Must Do Before National Health Insurance." *Medical Economics*, October 12, 1970.

———. "Multiphasic Health Testing and Medical Care as a Right." *New England Journal of Medicine* 283, no. 20 (November 12, 1970): 1087-9.

———. "New Trends in a Health Care System." Address to the AMA Symposium on Computer Systems in Medicine, Las Vegas, NV, February 16-17, 1971.

———. "Free Care Concept May Overload U.S. Health Services." *Geriatrics* 26, no. 4 (April 1971): 41 *passim*.

———. "An Ideal Nursing Unit." *Hospitals: Journal of the American Hospital Association* 45, no. 12 (June 16, 1971): 80-6.

———. "Prevention of Dissipation of Health Services Resources." *American Journal of Public Health* 61, no. 8 (August 1971): 1499-1506.

———. "A Clear Look at the Economics of Medical Care." Address to the symposium Technology and Health Care Systems in the 1980s, San Francisco, CA, January 19-21, 1972.

———. "Health Care and Health Services Resources." *Medical Progress Through Technology* 1, no. 1 (March 1972): 2-6.

———. "A New Medical Care Delivery System Model." In Proceedings of an International Conference on Health Technology Systems, San Francisco, CA, November 14-16, 1973.

———. "The Computer and New Health Care Systems." In *Hospital Computer Systems*. New York: John Wiley & Sons, 1974.

———. Interview by Daniella Thompson. Oakland, CA, 1974.

———. "Health Evaluation's Great Promise for Medical Care of the Future." Address, audience unknown, November 5, 1974.

———. "The Potential Opportunities of Systemized Prepaid Care." In *Health Handbook: An International Reference on Care and Cure*. Amsterdam: North-Holland Publishing Co., 1976.

———. "Evolving New Model for Health Care Delivery." *Orthopaedic Review* 5, no. 3 (March 1976): 19-21.

———. Remarks upon receiving an award from the American Planning Society at the American Hospital Association Annual Meeting, Anaheim, CA, August 26, 1977.

———. Remarks on receiving the Lyndon Baines Johnson Foundation Award, New York, October 27, 1977.

———. "Facilities Design and Construction." In *Multiphasic Health Testing Services*. New York: John Wiley & Sons, 1978.

———. Interview by Dan Scannell. Audio-video recording. Oakland, CA, 1978.

———. "Health of a Nation." Address at Riva de Gauda, Italy, April 1978.

———. "Health Testing – A New Concept of Health Care Delivery." In *Health Handbook: An International Reference on Care and Cure*. Amsterdam: North-Holland Publishing Co., 1979.

———. Address at WellCare Systems of the Future, Saltsjobaden, Sweden, May 1979.

———. Remarks on receiving an award from the American Association for Hospital Planning, August 25, 1979.

———. "A Rational Care Model for Health Care of a Nation." In *Lecture Notes in Medical Informatics: Technology and Health: Man and His World*. Berlin: Springer-Verlag, 1980.

———. Interview by Joan Trauner, Oakland, CA, not dated, c. 1981.

———. "50 Years With HMO's." *Private Practice*, April 1981.

———. Address to the 55th Annual Medical Group Management Association Conference, New Orleans, LA, October 13, 1981.

———. "Keynote Address to the IHEA '82: New Primary Care Delivery Systems." *Medical Informatics* 7, no. 3 (1982): 165-8.

———. Interview by Mimi Stein, Oakland, CA, February 17, 1982.

———. "The Coulee Dream: A Fond Remembrance of Edgar Kaiser." *KP Reporter*, January 1982.

———. Address on the subject of "Total Health Care" at Coto de Caza, CA, December 10, 1982.

———. "Worthy of Being Copied." Address to the Kaiser Family Foundation Board of Trustees, [Oakland, CA], June 26, 1983.

———. "The Delivery of Medical Care." *Scientific American* 222, no. 4 (April 1970): 15ff. Reprint, *M.D. Computing.* 11, no. 1 (Jan-Feb 1994): 43-7.

Garfield, Sidney R., Morris F. Collen, Robert Feldman, Krikor Soghikian, Robert H. Richart, and James H. Duncan. "Evaluation of an Ambulatory Medical-Care Delivery System." *New England Journal of Medicine* 294, no. 8 (February 19, 1976): 426-31.

Garfield, Sidney R., Cecil Cutting, Robert Feldman, Stephen Taller, and Morris F. Collen. *Total Health Care Project: Final Report. 2 vols.* Oakland, CA: Permanente Medical Group, Inc., 1987.

Garfield, Sidney, Cecil Cutting, and Morris Collen. "Historical Remarks Presented to the Executive Committee." Address delivered at the TPMG Executive Committee, Oakland, CA, April 24, 1974.

Garfield, Sidney R. and Clarence Mayhew. "The Modern Hospital of the Month: Walnut Creek Hospital; Efficiency Centers on the Corridor." *The Modern Hospital* 82 (March 1954): 61-72.

The Permanente Medical Group. *Manuscripts.* Kaiser Permanente Heritage Resources Archive, Oakland, CA.

Richart, Robert H., James H. Duncan, Sidney R. Garfield, and Morris F. Collen. "An Evaluation Model for Health Care System Change." *Journal of Medical Systems* 1 (1977): 65-77.

Weeks, Lewis, ed. *Sidney R. Garfield in First Person: An Oral History.* Hospital Administration Oral History Collection. Chicago: American Hospital Association, 1974.

❧ Index ❧

A Timeline of the Life of Sidney R. Garfield, M.D.

1906 – Sidney Roy Garfield is born in Elizabeth, New Jersey.

. . . .

1928 – Garfield earns his M.D. from the University of Iowa Medical School and completes a one-year internship.

. . . .

1929 – Garfield begins first residency training in general surgery at Los Angeles County General Hospital.

. . . .

1931 – Garfield begins a second, two-year residency program as Head Resident in Surgery at Los Angeles County General Hospital.

. . . .

1933 – Garfield opens a small, 12-bed hospital near Desert Center, California, to serve workers building the aqueduct bringing Colorado River water to Los Angeles.

. . . .

1934 – Garfield adds prepayment and accident prevention to his practice and is able to build and staff two additional hospitals for aqueduct workers.

. . . .

1938 – Edgar Kaiser, son of industrialist Henry J. Kaiser, convinces an initially reluctant Garfield to create a similar medical program for the workers building the Grand Coulee Dam in Washington.

. . . .

1939 – Garfield opens the Grand Coulee plan to workers' families and adds group medical practice, organizing all care "under one roof."

. . . .

1941 – With the U.S. entry into World War II, Henry J. Kaiser creates record-breaking shipbuilding operations in Richmond, California, and on the Columbia River in Portland, Oregon, and Vancouver, Washington, with steel produced in Fontana, California.

. . . .

1941 – Kaiser again calls on Garfield to create a medical care program. Within a year, he has built the largest civilian medical care program on the World War II Home Front.

. . . .

1945 – Garfield states that "maintenance of health" is the central mission of his program and attributes his success to combining prepayment, group practice, prevention, and facilities "under one roof." With Kaiser, he opens the medical care program to the public.

. . . .

1948 – At the height of opposition from the medical mainstream to Garfield's prepaid group practice model, he successfully defends himself against numerous charges brought before the Alameda-Contra Costa Medical Society to try to shut down his medical care program.

. . . .

1950 – Garfield's medical care program expands to tens of thousands of members when the West Coast International Longshoremen's and Warehousemen's Union joins, followed by 30,000 Retail Clerks Union members in Los Angeles within the year.

. . . .

1955 – The "Tahoe Agreement" resolves governance disputes among Permanente Medical Groups and the Kaiser Foundation Health Plan and Hospitals, though Garfield loses his leadership role and becomes vice president of facilities and planning.

. . . .

1960 – Garfield challenges Kaiser Permanente to find new methods of providing health care, rather than just sick care, by using emerging computer technology. He triggers a revolutionary research program that develops prototypical electronic medical records.

. . . .

1970 – Garfield publishes "The Delivery of Medical Care," the most important paper of his career, in *Scientific American*. It is a blueprint for the modern Kaiser Permanente.

. . . .

1984 – Sidney Garfield dies while working on his last research project — "Total Health" — which colleagues complete in 1987. Its name is the basis for the modern description Kaiser Permanente uses for itself — a "Total Health" organization.

. . . .